What the Experts Are Saying About *The Truth About Back Pain*

"This is the best work that I've read in quite some time concerning the treatment of back pain. It is easy to read and provides information that readers can implement immediately into their everyday lives. I have already incorporated some of Dr. Sinett's ideas into my own practice and my patients have seen the results."

—Peter Ottone, DC

"There are so many causes of back pain that unless a patient becomes more aware of what is causing his or her problem, it makes it difficult to help them remain pain-free. I will gladly recommend this book to my clients, as anything that helps them helps me."

—Rachel Williams, physical therapist

"It is refreshing to see that someone has looked at the interaction between diet and other aspects of our physiology. This book takes a thorough look at the connections between diet and back pain and offers a step-by-step, nutritionally sound approach to back pain relief."

—Stephanie Clarke, MSc, RD, and Willow Jarosh, MSc, RD

"Sit-ups and crunches have long been thought to be a necessary part of a good workout. *The Truth About Back Pain* showed me that when my next client asks for exercises that will give him or her a 'strong six-pack,' I'll teach some of the 'safe back' exercises recommended in this book."

—Eric von Frohlich, personal trainer

"The highest compliment I can give another professional is that of a patient referral. I send many of my patients who complain of neck and back pain to Dr. Sinett, because I know he'll be able to help them. His book is a great gift to back and neck pain sufferers because now he can help even more people."

—Louis Morledge, MD

continued…

"A must-read for anyone suffering from back pain."

—Maria Herrera, MD, physiatrist

"A good back program like the one in *The Truth About Back Pain* can make a big difference in people's lives."

—Jeff Silber, MD, orthopedic surgeon

"Finally an approachable and comprehensive guide to understanding the relationship between psychological and neurological pain that will be indispensable to the clinician and patient alike. . . . This groundbreaking work provides new understandings into the body-mind connection. As a psychotherapist I find that the principles in this book have allowed my patients to achieve the physical and emotional healing which we all seek."

—Leslie K. Bornstein, LCSW, BCD

The Truth About
BACK PAIN

A Revolutionary, Individualized Approach
to Diagnosing and Healing Back Pain

Todd Sinett, DC, and
Sheldon Sinett, DC

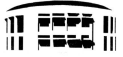
A PERIGEE BOOK

A PERIGEE BOOK
Published by the Penguin Group
Penguin Group (USA) Inc.
375 Hudson Street, New York, New York 10014, USA
Penguin Group (Canada), 90 Eglinton Avenue East, Suite 700, Toronto, Ontario M4P 2Y3, Canada (a division of Pearson
Penguin Canada Inc.) • Penguin Books Ltd., 80 Strand, London WC2R 0RL, England • Penguin Group Ireland, 25 St.
Stephen's Green, Dublin 2, Ireland (a division of Penguin Books Ltd.) • Penguin Group (Australia), 250 Camberwell Road,
Camberwell, Victoria 3124, Australia (a division of Pearson Australia Group Pty. Ltd.) • Penguin Books India Pvt. Ltd., 11
Community Centre, Panchsheel Park, New Delhi—110 017, India • Penguin Group (NZ), 67 Apollo Drive, Rosedale, North
Shore 0632, New Zealand (a division of Pearson New Zealand Ltd.) • Penguin Books (South Africa) (Pty.) Ltd., 24 Sturdee
Avenue, Rosebank, Johannesburg 2196, South Africa
Penguin Books Ltd., Registered Offices: 80 Strand, London WC2R 0RL, England

While the author has made every effort to provide accurate telephone numbers and Internet addresses at the time of
publication, neither the publisher nor the author assumes any responsibility for errors or for changes that occur after
publication. Further, the publisher does not have any control over and does not assume any responsibility for author or third-
party websites or their content.

PRINTING HISTORY
Perigee hardcover edition / March 2008
Perigee trade paperback edition / April 2009

Perigee trade paperback ISBN: 978-0-399-53485-0

The Library of Congress has cataloged the Perigee hardcover edition as follows:

Sinett, Todd.
   The truth about back pain : a revolutionary, individualized approach to diagnosing and healing back pain / Todd Sinett and
Sheldon Sinett.— 1st ed.
      p.   cm.
   Includes index.
   ISBN 978-0-399-53393-8
   1. Backache.   I. Sinett, Sheldon.   II. Title.
   RD771.B217S573 2008
   617.5'64—dc22   2007044269

PRINTED IN THE UNITED STATES OF AMERICA
10   9   8   7   6   5   4   3   2

PUBLISHER'S NOTE: Neither the publisher nor the author is engaged in rendering professional advice or services to the individual reader. The ideas, procedures, and suggestions contained in this book are not intended as a substitute for consulting
with your physician. All matters regarding your health require medical supervision. Neither the author nor the publisher shall
be liable or responsible for any loss or damage allegedly arising from any information or suggestion in this book. The recipes
contained in this book are to be followed exactly as written. The publisher is not responsible for your specific health or aller-
gy needs that may require medical supervision. The publisher is not responsible for any adverse reactions to the recipes contained in this book.

This book is dedicated to the most wonderful father a son could ever have.

I joined my father's chiropractic office in 1995. As the practice thrived and became a truly holistic center for healing, we grew determined to share what we had learned by way of a book for a larger audience. Unfortunately, during the period we were working on the book, my dad died of complications following heart surgery. Finishing it alone was one of the hardest things I have ever done, but it was very important to him—to both of us—to share our philosophy, because we both believed it could help many thousands of people suffering with back pain.

The best compliment I get is when someone says I am just like my father. He lived a regret-free life filled with love. He was a ray of sunshine with a magnetic personality, whose main interest was in helping others. He had so much vitality, it was often said that his energy had energy. When people asked how old my dad was, it was always a tricky question. He may have been chronologically 69 years old, but he had the exuberance of a 15-year-old kid. My mom said that for every day he lived, he actually lived a day and a half. So I suppose that would have made him 103.

Doctor in Latin means "to teach," and I want to thank him for teaching me how to be not only a doctor but also a father, husband, and friend. The time that we got to work together was the most special of my life. I miss my dad terribly, but I'm grateful that he left me a good instruction manual for carrying on his good works.

If my father were alive today, he would want to sincerely thank you for purchasing this book. And I am sure he would urge you to buy a couple extra copies because they make great gifts.

Contents

PART FOUR

It's All in Your Head: The Emotions and Back Pain

Introduction

You are reading this book because you or a loved one is suffering from back pain. You are far from alone. At some point in our lives, 85 percent of us will suffer back pain. It can even happen to people who specialize in helping relieve the back pain of others—I know, because it happened to my dad; and it was one of the toughest times in my family's history. Here is my father's story:

In the late 1950s, it was suggested to me that becoming a chiropractor would be a promising profession that would provide a hands-on way of helping and healing people. I decided to pursue an education in the field, graduating in 1963. To save money on rent when I was getting started, I opened my practice in my mother's living room in Brooklyn, New York. I would see patients, and they would leave the apartment, feeling better after treatment and fortified with a gift of baked goods from my mother. Because of the strong intergenerational community connections we had, the practice became successful quite quickly. Soon I needed real office space, and I rented an office in Brooklyn, eventually buying the building.

Charging $10 for three treatments, I worked from 7:00 in the morning to 7:00 at night to try to fit in as many patients as I could because I saw that hands-on chiropractic medicine was making a big difference in people's lives.

I always loved my work, but I treasured my free time, too. One of my weekend pleasures has always been a good game of tennis. I used to play a lot, but one day I bent down to pick up a tennis ball, and I was unable to stand up again because of severe lower back pain! My back spasms were so painful that I spent the next 9 months lying flat in bed. As a chiropractor, my first instinct was to turn to fellow professionals. When that didn't help, I started working my way through physical therapists, orthopedists, acupuncturists, and neurologists. No one could get to the bottom of my unrelenting back spasms. I felt absolutely terrible. I could not work; my patients were having to turn elsewhere for help, and my practice was diminishing dramatically. My family and I were desperate—if we had heard of a shaman in Nepal who could have helped me, I think we would have gone! Then an orthopedic surgeon finally suggested "exploratory surgery," meaning that he would open me up to "look around for a possible cause." That was it for me. I became frantic to find another solution.

Not knowing where else to turn, I thought back to a course I had taken from a chiropractor with the fortunate name of George Goodheart. Goodheart, then working in Detroit, Michigan, had created a new technique called Applied Kinesiology, and I put myself on his monthlong waiting list for an appointment. It was Goodheart who finally helped me banish my back pain. Though I had been poked and prodded and tested and examined in almost every way imaginable, Goodheart paid attention to me as a complete person. Although the other professionals did what they could in pursuit of curing the hurt, Goodheart took a step back and asked, "Why?" Like a good detective, he looked into my past for a cause. He asked about my life and my lifestyle, and he scrutinized everything from what I ate to how angry I was about being incapacitated.

Within 2 short weeks of reconnecting with him, I was beginning to show my first signs of improvement, and I regained strength and health steadily from there. After studying what was going on throughout my body, Goodheart identified a cause: It was not my spine, it was not a slipped disc, it was not bad posture, it was not all in my head—my back pain actually stemmed from poor dietary habits. (You'll read more about this and some other surprising causes of back pain later in the book.) Once Goodheart understood the cause, he was able to develop a proper solution—which, in my case, involved reducing my heavily caffeinated, sugar-consuming ways. Suffice it to say, Goodheart basically saved my life. Without his intervention, I don't know when or if I would have gotten better.

Despite my profession, I am a classic example of how years of lifestyle and health imbalance can lead to severe back pain and dysfunction. Based on this experience, I resolved that I was going to take a new look at what Goodheart had taught me and see how I could apply that to my own work with my own patients. Goodheart's underlying message—that the body speaks a language that we need to learn and listen to—became a key element of my practice. I learned the importance of letting a patient's body explain the why of the back pain (and never assuming that the location of the pain necessarily indicated the true area of the problem).

Working with this new approach from the mid-1970s forward, I soon found that I was swamped with patients. Limousines were bringing patients from Manhattan to my office in Brooklyn, and it made good business sense for me to move my practice to New York City. In a very short period of time, I had one of the busiest chiropractic practices in the city.

Over the last 40 years, I have had the opportunity to refine my thinking about helping people with "what ails them." My son, Todd, joined me in 1995, and together we have worked to expand on this integrated approach to back pain that takes into account both the search for the why of the pain and the examination of what we've determined are the three vital components—structural, chemical (dietary), and emotional—of good health. Each of these factors needs to be carefully evaluated in order to come up with the right solution for a patient's pain, and that's what *The Truth About Back Pain* is about.

My intention is to provide you with a system that can be used to self-diagnose the possible root of your back pain; as a result, you will be able to find a solution much faster than my father did.

You'll read more about why a correct solution for back pain eludes most professionals, but for now what you need to remember is that professionals make two major mistakes when diagnosing back pain. First, they focus too closely on the location of the problem, which often has nothing to do with the cause of the pain (and, therefore, is not going to provide clues for a solution). Second, they forget about the interrelationship of all the body's systems. Back pain is sometimes caused by a combination of issues, so the doctor may recommend a fix for the issue that falls within his or her realm but that may still leave the patient coping with pain that is partially caused by something else.

Equally important, *The Truth About Back Pain* will make you a better partner in your own recovery. We already know that patients can be very intuitive about what may be the root cause of their pain. They sometimes just need help articulating the problem and working with their healthcare professional to find the best solution. Once you go through the diagnostic process that is laid out in this book, you'll see how important your role in your back health can be.

Why the Current System Fails Back Pain Sufferers

Unfortunately, you have not been getting the truth when it comes to getting rid of your back problem. Just as my father wasted months dealing with his own pain, back pain sufferers from all walks of life are being led down the wrong path. Because diagnosing back pain is a difficult and time-consuming process, many doctors have helped encourage the thought that having back pain is a normal progression of life.

I am here to tell you that it is not. I often tell patients that the advice they've gotten is a half truth because most of the time they are getting only a small portion of the diagnostic and therapeutic options. Each doctor brings to the situation a background from a particular specialty; as a result, he or she is not prepared to look at all of the possible causes of your back problem. Each doctor sees only a small percentage of the possible solutions because he or she bases the treatment on a very small piece of information.

Although doctors are well intentioned, our segmenting of health professionals by specialty works against the patient in areas such as back pain, which requires a broader perspective and an interdisciplinary approach. Only by stepping back to evaluate the whole person and the *why* of the problem can an effective treatment be found. This approach is often the only means by which some people are able to rid themselves of their back problem.

In *The Truth About Back Pain*, I present the whole truth and nothing but the truth. Throughout the book, the solutions to back pain are each clearly presented. But, like the many causes of back pain, there are many remedies, and not all will apply to you. It is my hope that other healthcare professionals who read this book will join me in the quest to change the treatment for back pain.

Who We Are

My late father, Sheldon Sinett, and I have devoted more than 50 years in chiropractic practice to treating people who suffer from back and neck pain. The practice my father established, and which I joined in 1995, in New York City includes other chiropractors as well as professionals who specialize in acupuncture, physical therapy, and nutrition. We've learned that to help people, we need to be able to offer options based on the root cause of their pain. Once the cause is known—whether it is structural, chemical, or emotional, or a combination of these—then the solution becomes clear.

My patient base consists of many different types of people of all ages and walks of life. Because our approach to healing works, we've been asked to treat a variety of luminaries from all over the world—including royals. (It's a little intimidating to treat someone whose bodyguard and personal physician won't leave the examining room!) Partly because New York City is such an entertainment hub, we are frequently called to come backstage at Madison Square Garden or at Broadway theaters when performers are in pain. Athletes—ranging from Major League Baseball players and U.S. Open tennis players—have also sought our help. Suffice it to say, we've seen it all. From the problems of the carpenter to the aches of the chorus dancer, our methods permit people to become pain-free.

Constant Learning Is Our Mantra

"The more you know, the more you find out how little you know," my father used to say. In our office, we are continually learning, trying to discover new information about what has an impact on back pain and develop new treatments. With this book, I am able to present you with a flexible and workable system that I know can help you with your back problem. I share with you your goal of correcting your back problem.

How to Use This Book

Many self-help books suggest that you start with the section that interests you most, but I can't say that with this book. First, you need to understand the basics—the information presented in Part I of the book. If you skip ahead to a section you think applies particularly to your situation, then you'll be missing an essential element of our approach to healing. Like so many well-intentioned doctors and patients, you'll be taking a narrow focus and possibly ignoring some vital piece of information that is a key to your recovery. You need to start at the beginning and read through the entire first section. By reading Chapters 1 to 3— which really can be done by most people in about an hour—you'll come to understand why you've had so much trouble finding relief for your back pain.

Once you complete the self-diagnostic questions in Chapter 3, you can *then* skip around and explore various sections of the book. I definitely want you to find relief at the earliest opportunity, so after you've read about our basic philosophy, turn to the section that seems most appropriate to you. Later on, however, come back to the book and go through the other sections—they are all interrelated.

Part II focuses on structural issues concerning back health and explains how your back and back muscles work. Everyone will benefit particularly from Chapter 6, which discusses core imbalance—a modern-day malady from which virtually all of us suffer.

Part III tackles the issue of chemical imbalances in the body caused by diet, digestion, and hormones. The emphasis here happens to be on improving your eating habits, which was my father's main problem and one that he shared with thousands of other sufferers. Although I would never refer to this dietary plan as a weight-loss diet, I can assure you that people who eat carefully and sensibly will, indeed, lose weight. You will also have more energy, feel better, and experience less stress. Good eating habits matter to overall health and have specific relevance to back pain, which few practitioners address.

Part IV examines the emotional causes of back pain, including stress. In this day and age, who can't benefit from some good suggestions on ways to get rid of emotional tension? This section offers everything from lessons learned from tai chi to the value of acupuncture to some basic do-at-your-desk stress-relieving exercises.

PART ONE

In the Beginning, There Is Back Pain

CHAPTER 1

Your Aching Back

If your back hurts, you are not alone. You suffer from one of the most common but vexing conditions of modern times. Back pain is so much a part of our culture that people seem to think this discomfort is simply part of daily life. For some people, back pain is debilitating, and they find it difficult, if not impossible, to get through each day. For others, the discomfort may be more like a nagging annoyance, but one that leads them to take ibuprofen or prescription painkillers in some quantity.

Here are some shocking statistics about back pain:

- Back pain sends more patients to physicians than any ailment except the common cold, and it accounts for a quarter of all workers' compensation claims.

- One-third of people over the age of 18 have sought treatment in the past 5 years for back pain.

- Back pain is the leading cause of job disability in adults younger than 45 years.

- The healthcare system spends more than $90 billion annually on back pain treatments—much of that for X-rays, computed tomography (CT) scans, injections, and surgeries, which studies show are often premature or unnecessary.

- As many as 4 in 10 imaging studies associated with lower back pain are unnecessary, and as many as two in three epidural steroid injections are avoidable, according to the National Committee for Quality Assurance, an organization that monitors healthcare quality and accredits health plans.

- According to the National Institutes of Health (NIH), back pain is the fifth most common reason for hospitalization and the third most common reason for surgery.

Help Me Make This Pain Go Away!

I know that statistics are the last thing you want to hear about right now—your aching back is pretty much all you can think about at this time. And while I will discuss the "what you should do" suggestions quite soon, first I want to explain what's meaningful and what isn't when it comes to back pain.

My favorite myths about back pain vividly illustrate why your confusion is so understandable—you've been hearing a lot of misinformation, ranging from medical misconceptions (imaging studies are helpful for making a diagnosis) to old wives' tales (if you are middle-aged, it's normal to have back pain).

Realizing that the following popular myths aren't always true will put you on the path toward better understanding.

Ten Myths About Back Pain

Myth 1: If you bend down to lift something up and your back goes out, it is because you bent wrong.

Very rarely will your back go out after you've made a simple movement, such as bending. If you suffer sudden back pain as a result of bending, it is more likely that you have been doing something that has damaged your back little by little. Bending was simply the final indignity, and your back responded with, "No more!"

Myth 2: The location of the back pain determines the problem.

The fact is, you may be experiencing pain in one part of the body but the problem often does not originate from the same spot. For example, an imbalance in your feet can cause your lower back to hurt.

Myth 3: Extra weight can be the primary cause of back pain.

While extra weight is not good for your body overall, your spine is not going to give out because of a few extra pounds. Being overweight is only one piece of the back pain puzzle—it is by no means the determining factor.

The question I always ask is, "Was the patient overweight before he or she had the back problem?" Extra weight is generally not the root problem; the unhealthy habits that caused the patient to be overweight in the first place are usually the primary reason for their back pain.

Myth 4: If you have back pain more than once, you will probably need to have surgery at some point.

Surgery is not inevitable; nothing could be further from the truth. It is always best to start with the least invasive solution. Back surgery is *not* a cure-all. The common model that the surgeon may present to you—that a disc sitting on a nerve needs to be corrected—is oversimplified and at best only partially true. As a rule of thumb, don't even consider surgery initially. It is not recommended during the first 6 weeks of pain onset; half of patients with radiating lower back pain recover spontaneously with pain management, minimal bed rest, and a return to appropriate physical activity.

According to the National Committee for Quality Assurance, patients often undergo aggressive treatments when less costly and less complicated therapy may yield similar or better results. Unfortunately, some patients who have back surgery find themselves suffering from failed back surgery syndrome (FBSS). The fact that there is actually a term to describe this situation says it all.

For a select few, back surgery can be the best course of action, but explore the less invasive solutions first.

Myth 5: MRIs are helpful for diagnosing back pain.

Magnetic resonance imaging (MRI) is actually ineffective when it comes to the diagnosis of back pain. Based on studies conducted between 1998 and 2000, doctors at the University of Washington in Seattle concluded that using MRIs leads to a higher rate of specialist consultations and more surgeries for patients, but results in fewer beneficial outcomes. In the *Journal of the American Medical Association*, Nortin M. Hadler, professor of medicine at the University of North Carolina at Chapel Hill, noted that MRIs are not effective for patients with back pain because the imagery is insufficient to diagnose the root cause.

Myth 6: The best way to predict future occurrences of back pain is with an X-ray and/or blood work.

In one study, 3,000 Boeing employees were followed over a period of 4 years. The investigators found that psychological stress was a far more accurate predictor of future back pain problems than any physical measure.

Myth 7: By age 60, it is normal to have some back pain in the morning.

It is not normal, but it is very common for middle-aged adults to experience back pain. However, back pain does not have to be a life sentence that worsens as you age.

Myth 8: If you have a disc herniation, there is nothing that you can do; you just have to learn to live with pain.

There are thousands of people who have a disc herniation who have absolutely *no symptoms.* In a landmark study published in the *New England Journal of Medicine*, researchers found that 28 percent of the people whose MRI results revealed a disc herniation have actually never suffered back pain.

Myth 9: To have a strong back, you need strong abdominals and a strong core; the best way to achieve this is through sit-ups and crunches.

Sit-ups and crunches actually cause more back pain than they prevent. I've treated so many patients who have hurt themselves by doing these exercises that I am perfectly willing to tell you that these can be the worst exercises you can do.

Yes, you want to strengthen your back by having a well-functioning core and abdominals, but the abdominal exercises (like sit-ups) that doctors have been recommending for years have nothing to do with stabilizing your back because they work the wrong abdominal muscles. The ideal exercise for back strengthening is an exercise called "The Skinnies" (see Chapter 6), which works a small internal abdominal muscle called the transverse abdominus.

Myth 10: Diet has nothing to do with back pain.
"You are what you eat" happens to be true about back pain. When people digest food, they have a *viscerosomatic reaction*. This means that as the digestive system processes the food, it can affect the muscles. Just as every joint and muscle seems to ache if you have an alcohol-induced hangover, the same type of viscerosomatic reaction occurs when you eat foods that disagree with you in some way.

An Urgent Message from Your Body (and What Happens Next)

"My back hurts" sounds like a simple complaint, but it's actually your body pleading for attention. Patients often come to me with guesses as to what caused their pain, based on what they, or their doctors, might know to be factors of back pain, such as:

- Trauma or injury; fracture

- Degeneration of a vertebra

- Protruding disc

- Ligament or muscle tears

- Muscle tension

- Overuse (back strain) or improper exercise

- Poor muscle tone

- Back-related joint problems

- Infection and tumors. Spinal column infections and tumors are not common and, unfortunately, both conditions are difficult to diagnose. Because they are potentially quite serious, physicians sometimes spend a lot of time exploring this possibility when nothing else seems likely.

- Obesity

- Hormone issues

- Smoking. A smoker's risk of lower back pain is actually 1.5 to 2.5 times greater than that of a nonsmoker. Nicotine may impair the availability of nutrients to the discs. (This is just one more reason people should quit smoking; for more, see Part III.)

Once a cause is determined, the logical treatment options follow, with varying degrees of effectiveness:

- **ACTIVITY MODIFICATION**. Cutting back on some of your physical activities can be a tolerable option early on, but this "solution" causes additional problems if you have to modify your activity for more than a few days. If you withdraw from activities for a prolonged period of time, then muscles weaken; furthermore, this leads many people to become slightly depressed. This is truly counterproductive.

- **MEDICATION**. It can be helpful briefly for acute pain.

- **PHYSICAL REHABILITATION OR THERAPY**. If the diagnosis is complete and the cause is understood, this is a good option.

- **OCCUPATIONAL THERAPY**. Like physical rehabilitation or therapy, this can be a very good option.

- **IMPROVED BACK SUPPORT AT THE OFFICE**. People often notice their pain during or after long days sitting at the computer terminal. Ergonomic seating and a better workstation setup can certainly help but is rarely a cure-all.

- **WEIGHT LOSS**. This is a good idea for many reasons, but lots of thin people have back pain. Weight loss is by no means a cure-all of any kind.

- **SMOKING CESSATION.** Though this is a great idea, it's a hard sell to most people, who often smoke *more* during bouts of back pain.

- **BACK PAIN PREVENTION PROGRAM.** This is another good idea, but unless the true cause has been diagnosed, one has to ask, "Prevent what?" Is the person suffering back pain because of a structural problem? Is there an emotional root to the problem? Until a correct diagnosis is made, there is no way to start a back pain prevention program; a solution cannot be sought if the cause hasn't been found.

- **ASSISTIVE DEVICES OR MECHANICAL BACK SUPPORTS.** This can be helpful for acute pain, but devices can create dependence, which can lead to future muscle weakness and more pain.

- **SURGERY.** It is important when absolutely necessary, but exploratory surgery should be avoided at all costs. Back surgery is not a cure-all, but for issues such as disc herniation and spinal stenosis, surgery can be a solution. However, if you do not have proof that you have one of these conditions, then exhaust all other options before going under the knife.

As you read this book, you'll learn to separate the myths from the facts, and you'll soon understand the truth about back pain. If you're like most of our patients, you've seen your regular doctor and a specialist or two—and you've been sent for an X-ray or an MRI or maybe both. You may have tried painkillers, bed rest, health-food-store remedies, elixirs, and exercises, but you're still suffering. I hear and see this situation every day, but I have an idea as to why so much of what is done has thus far been ineffective against back pain.

What's Wrong with Our System

Many doctors owe you an apology. If we were talking football instead of back pain, the win–loss record for the medical profession's fight against back pain would definitely merit the immediate removal of the coach and all of the team's players. Yet we go on with the same futile approach to back pain.

Today's standard approach is based on searching for the pathological condition of the back itself. The assumption is that the person has a structural problem, so the doctor will perform a physical examination; do some blood work; and perhaps order X-rays or an MRI study if he or she suspects a slipped disc, a crushed vertebra, or some other structural cause for the pain.

Back pain is an equal opportunity disorder. It occurs in people of all ages, of both genders, and who do all types of work—from hard labor to desk work. You would think someone in the government or at a top-notch teaching hospital would have put together a blue-ribbon panel of experts from different fields to examine causes and cures of back pain. Unfortunately, however, when it comes to back pain, everyone has an idea of what ought to be done, but no one seems to have a true solution.

A Blue-Ribbon Test That Makes Me Blue

Very often modern technology, such as MRI, is used to help doctors find an abnormality. This type of testing is so commonly used that many patients come into the office and demand that we send them for an MRI study, "because that's what my coworker or friend had." The thinking goes that a disc or bone is pressing on a nerve root, so the MRI study can be used to observe what is happening to the nerve. These structural malformations provide the evidence on which medical professionals base their structural theories and treatments.

However, there are many studies that refute these theories. In 1994, researchers reported a controlled study, published in the *New England Journal of Medicine*, in which MRI studies were conducted on 98 people who were symptom-free of back pain. Almost two-thirds (64 percent) of these people showed clear evidence of a bulging or protruding disc, and 28 percent showed disc herniation—the type of a spinal abnormalities that would seem to indicate severe back ailments. Yet these people did not suffer from any type of back pain whatsoever. Based on this evidence, the idea of diagnosing solely from an MRI is clearly misguided.

Another study verified that the use of MRI studies is unnecessary. A controlled randomized trial described in the June 2003 issue of the *Journal of the*

American Medical Association showed that X-rays were better than MRIs for diagnosing issues for most patients who suffered lower back pain. Radiographs actually led to fewer interventions and ultimately fewer surgeries. While an X-ray is less sensitive than an MRI, it shows what is relevant to back pain. With back pain, less can be more.

It is easy to see the appeal of an MRI, said Stanley J. Bigos, professor emeritus of orthopedic surgery and environmental health at the University of Washington. "The reality is patients want an answer, the doctor wants to get the patient out of the room and the hypotheses start to flow."

Imaging (X-ray, MRI, CT) serves only to bolster the notion that back pain is nothing more than the symptom of an underlying disease. Many conventional physicians and surgeons miss the true underlying causes of back pain because they continue to be stuck on the easy explanation offered by high-tech imaging. All too often, the orthopedist who sees a herniated disc on an MRI decides that the only answer is surgery: If the problem is a herniation, the remedy is simple: Fix the disc!

When no structural abnormality is found, patients are sent off with a pat on the shoulder and a prescription for anti-inflammatory or other types of painkilling drugs to make them feel better. Painkillers are not real solutions (more about that later in the chapter), let alone cures; they merely mask the pain. Giving a painkiller to relieve back pain is a little like taking the battery out of a smoke alarm because the noise is too loud. Although pain relievers may be necessary as part of the overall diagnosis and treatment, you need to put out the fire, not just deal with the loudness of the alarm.

Because the traditional medical profession has no real answers, back pain sufferers turn to all types of alternatives. Think about the number of cures—from twisting and stretching machines to herbal remedies—you've seen talked about on cable television stations and the Internet. But these options aren't the answer, either.

There's Nothing Structurally Wrong . . .

When doctors get to the head-scratching phase—after X-rays, after MRI studies, after blood work, and after other testing—they sometimes determine that the problem is emotional, often implying that it's all in your head.

Patients then come to me, saying: "The doctor tested me for everything, and it all came out negative. He says it's all in my head." For a time, this concept was viewed as revolutionary because it challenged the status quo. The people who promoted the emotional argument bolstered their case by pointing out that the structural fixes don't work, so this *must* be the answer. Unfortunately, this approach is not the missing answer, either.

As you'll read in Part IV, sometimes our emotions are at the root of our pain. But the problem with this as a possible cause for back pain often has to do with the way it is presented: Patients are often made to feel that the pain is something they made up or *imagined*. They come to my office feeling guilty and in despair because, indeed, they find themselves flat on their back in bed every time the in-laws show up. Although the cause of the problem may be emotional, the reaction is very physical. Your in-laws show up and your back muscles tighten so much you can't move; that's not your fault, and there are very clear ways to get those muscles to loosen up. While we probably won't be able to keep your in-laws from visiting, we *will* be able to keep you up and active despite an impending family visit.

Do Nothing . . . Wait and See

For many physicians, when no cause is clear, they rightly fear that the potential solutions may be worse than the original problem. In a 2004 article in the *New York Times*, Dr. Nortin Hadler is quoted as saying, "Today individuals with regional back pain might fare less poorly by managing as best they can on their own, perhaps with some lay advice, than if they chose to become primary care patients."

A variety of studies have suggested that in 85 percent of cases it is impossible to say why a person's back hurts, says Richard Deyo, professor of medicine and health services at the University of Washington. That's the crux of the problem—the medical community as a whole doesn't really understand the probable causes of back pain.

For people with chronic pain, some doctors are now advocating a different approach altogether: teaching people to live with pain, to put aside the understandable fear that any motion will aggravate their injury.

On one level, I certainly commend this approach, because these healthcare professionals are applying the very important doctrine of "First, do no harm." Unfortunately, many people who follow this advice have been dealing with discomfort for so long that they have become experts at managing their lives around pain. They have become contortionists—sitting, standing, and sleeping in pain-avoidance positions that are not good for their spines. Had they realized that help was available, they could have worked toward a solution much sooner.

Back pain is one of the most debilitating health issues facing people in the United States. How's this for a summary of where medical professionals are in terms of helping people: *A large majority of people have back pain, and we don't know why. Therefore, we must ask: How can it be cured? The answer is quite simple: It can't, but we sure have invested a lot of money and technology in trying.*

Pretty discouraging, isn't it? We know how desperate people are for relief, and that's why we've worked hard to develop solutions.

The Harm Is Even Deeper Than You Might Think

Although the inability to find an answer to your back pain is a sorry state of affairs, the current approach is actually harmful: People are given little hope for getting better, and this alone—a diagnosis with no solution—is debilitating. (Insurance companies insist on a diagnosis, so whether or not the doctor treating you fully understands what is going on with your back, he or she is forced by the system to write something down.)

Doctors are trained to make a diagnosis, spending thousands of hours trying to hone their skills to name a condition. We expect to go to the doctor and have him or her tell us what the problem is and how to fix it. However, determining the cause of pain and then treating it is quite complex, and most physicians have a limited amount of time to spend with each patient. As a result, there is a tendency to focus on the *most likely* cause of the problem. Patients often leave with the impression that their initial diagnosis is also their *final* diagnosis.

The difficulty of being labeled with a disease was brought home to me when

I was a child. When I was 8 years old, my father discovered that I had swollen glands, so off to the doctor we went. After a physical examination, blood work, and urinalysis, the doctor diagnosed me with idiopathic lymphadenopathy.

Holy cow! I had *idiopathic lymphadenopathy*!

I was prescribed an antibiotic to treat this serious condition. The antibiotic never helped, but fortunately for me, the swollen glands eventually went away. I have since gotten numerous examinations, none of which has revealed any lasting effects of my earlier condition.

It wasn't until I was studying to become a doctor that I discovered what idiopathic lymphadenopathy was: *Idiopathic* means "unknown origin," and *lymphadenopathy* means "swollen glands." So my diagnosis had been that I had swollen glands but the doctor didn't know why.

Two unfortunate things happened as a result of the doctor's need to label my condition: He prescribed an antibiotic for no apparent reason, and he felt he had to sound intelligent by hiding behind language rather than just saying that I had swollen glands but he didn't know why.

The medical community has created a whole language that justifies people having back pain. We use terms such as *degenerative disc disease*, *osteoarthritis*, and *spinal stenosis*, and there are countless theories as to what to do about each.

Unfortunately, these terms aren't so different from a witch doctor's spell. The villager finds out that the witch doctor has cast a spell of death over him and that he has 2 days to live. Everyone believes in the power of the witch doctor so, lo and behold, the person dies within 2 days. These fear diagnoses sometimes place a patient in a mind-set to jump into a promised cure too quickly or cause others to delay treatment. Because a label has been placed on what these patients have, they sometimes feel they just have to endure.

It's time to rethink the way health practitioners deal with this type of serious discomfort and come up with a more effective solution.

If I were to wish only one thing for my patients, it would be for them to learn to listen to their bodies. If your back hurts, your body is giving very clear signals that something is wrong, and it's time to pay attention. If no one takes time to understand the underlying cause of the pain, it's all but impossible to banish the problem—that's why we have a nation of back pain sufferers.

Not Enough Why

"Too much what and not enough why" is the way my dad came to describe the problem of creating a diagnosis without understanding the underlying cause. I know this phrase sounds like part of an Abbott and Costello routine, but it clearly describes the crux of our healthcare problem.

If doctors were trained in the pursuit of why, we would be better off. *Why* is a person having an arthritic type reaction in his joints? Could it be a nutritional deficiency, an allergic reaction, or the result of a poor diet? Or *why* is a person having neck pain every single day except Sundays? Her lifestyle is likely to offer an explanation. The why is key.

Most healthcare professionals are well trained in the what when it comes to diagnosing and treating illness, but it is the pursuit of the why that leads to a completely different set of solutions.

Over the last few decades, we've been refining the method my father hit upon as a result of his own bout with back pain (see page ix for his story). He eventually found relief for his pain and, in the process, adopted an analytical approach that there are three possible causes of back pain:

- **STRUCTURAL**. A postural issue; something such as muscle or bone out of alignment.

- **CHEMICAL**. Diet can actually be at the root of some types of pain.

- **EMOTIONAL**. Muscle tension due to stress.

These are the three major points underlying the healing philosophy in this book: a unique, integrated, holistic method for banishing pain.

The system outlined here is one that was originally created by a fellow chiropractor, George Goodheart, whose studies of kinesiology (the study of the anatomy, physiology, and mechanics of body movement) led him to create the system he used to help my father. Over time, my father fine-tuned this method into the program that we've employed since the 1970s. We have learned that the most important thing we need to determine is the *reason* for the pain; then, and only then, can a proper treatment be developed.

The Power of Listening

One day a patient asked me what made our practice so successful. I answered with some self-deprecating humor, noting that I thought people came for the fruit we always have available. (My grandmother taught my dad that when you welcome a patient into the office, you should act as if he or she were a guest in your home.) The patient chuckled at my response, but the question stuck in my head for the remainder of the day.

A back problem is not just a back problem; it's a health issue. Pain is a language we know, and most of the time back pain is caused by a couple of different factors. Our success is based on our actions: We ask, we listen, and we follow leads that benefit our patients. We've been able to help countless people overcome their back pain. In the process, we have helped people achieve an overall improvement in their general well-being.

Once you understand the cause, you'll be able to evaluate your situation and determine what aspects of your life you can alter on your own. You will learn about how your posture, your work environment, your exercise practices, your stress level, and your diet affect your back health. And if a professional is needed to help you get over a final difficulty, we'll help you evaluate the healthcare professional you may choose to consult.

Wonderful Vs. Bullshit

I'll close this chapter with a story about what is happening in our healthcare system today. Patients, armed with the best-guess diagnoses from professionals, come into our office telling us exactly what they think is happening and what needs to be done. Then they'll let us know what their own doctor says they should do. These encounters, which happen many times a week, remind me of a story that I am fond of recounting:

Three elderly women are sitting on a park bench discussing how wonderful their sons are. One lady says, "My son is so wonderful that he sends me on a trip around the world for my birthday every year."

"Wonderful," says the third lady, while the second one explains that her son is so wonderful that he buys her a new car every year; she barely drives it, but she accepts it anyway.

The third woman again says, "Wonderful!" So the first two women ask her, "So what does your son get you?"

The woman replies that her son sent her to charm school for her birthday.

"Charm school?" say the other two in surprise.

"Yes, charm school," she says. "In charm school we learned to say 'wonderful' instead of 'bullshit.'"

Unfortunately, I see far too many patients who are getting "wonderful" diagnoses. Chapter 2 reveals a brand-new world to you, introducing our three-tiered approach and integrated treatment philosophy. It is the method that worked for my father and for countless patients we've seen since, and we know it will work for you, too. And that's no BS.

The Back Pain Solution

Christopher Columbus set sail from Spain in search of a quicker travel route to Asia. Though he was armed with mileage calculations and the best maps of the day, he ran into a major obstacle on his way: the Americas.

Just as Columbus was never going to get to the East Indies with an inaccurate map, we face the same problem with our current approach to back pain. Essentially, we are making the same mistake Christopher Columbus did. We are basing our diagnoses and treatments on erroneous information. We have been working with the wrong map for back pain, and it's never going to get us where we need to go.

A New Approach to Back Pain

When patients arrive in our offices, the diagnosis they have received is usually partially true. Most doctors utilize the clearest imaging technology (often an MRI) to diagnose the problem. They usually look for a structural cause, which certainly makes sense initially, and then they recommend anti-inflammatory medications, muscle relaxants, home exercises, physical therapy, and, if none of those things work, surgery.

As you read in Chapter 1, the search for a structural issue is problematic, because back abnormalities *may or may not* cause pain. Yes, a patient may have a slight structural abnormality, but that may not actually be at the root of the pain. Recall the 1994 study, which I cited previously, in which almost two-thirds of the people whose MRIs showed evidence of structural back abnormalities suffered no pain at all. Because so many people *do* suffer back pain—with or without structural abnormalities—we obviously need a new diagnostic method.

This chapter explains our three-tiered approach to back pain. We have used it with thousands of patients, and it has proved to us that imbalance in any one of the following three areas may contribute to or cause pain:

- **STRUCTURAL PROBLEMS** involving bones, muscles, and nerves

- **CHEMICAL ACTIONS** related to hormonal and digestive issues that affect the body on a chemical and cellular level

- **EMOTIONAL STRESS**, or the psychological factors that lead to imbalance in the musculoskeletal, nervous, hormonal, and immune systems

Back Pain Isn't Really the Problem

You read that right—it is my belief that back pain itself is not the problem! Back pain is only a symptom of the real trouble. Pain is the body's way of trying to protect you from doing further damage to your body. The medical community spends its time and research money trying to get rid of the pain, when we should instead be looking for the true causes of back problems.

Imagine, for example, that you bend over to retrieve a tennis ball, or stoop to pick up some dirty laundry. You hear an odd, cracking sound. As you try to stand up, you feel a sharp, knife-like cramp in the small of your back. The back pain you experience is not random. It is a reliable and predictable symptom of something else that is happening in your body, and the pain is a signal. You are being given the opportunity to remedy the situation before it becomes more serious.

As discussed in Chapter 1, instead of asking "Where does it hurt?" we need to start asking "*Why* does it hurt?" Whether the principal cause is structural (muscles and bones), chemical (nutrition and hormonal), or emotional (stress related), these imbalances are all interrelated. We often find that the problem stems from a combination of two of these issues, and sometimes all three.

Do you have a herniated disc? Possibly. But the real cause of your pain may be the three cups of coffee you drink daily. Or the actual trigger may be the distress you feel about a situation with a loved one. "It feels like someone jabbing a sword into my back," said one patient about the anguish he felt during his divorce.

Remember, too, that back pain is rarely one catastrophic event but several situations combining to create back pain (like the winds gathering to create a perfect storm). Any one of these factors, or a combination thereof, can be the one that catapults you into unbearable agony.

In Chapter 3 we walk you through a self-diagnostic program that will help you understand what might be at the root of *your* back pain, but first it's important to understand how the three possible causes of back pain can affect you.

Structural Causes of Back Pain

"Look first to the spine for the cause of disease," said Hippocrates. We couldn't agree more. If your back hurts, then checking for a structural cause is a good place to start.

The first structural issue to consider, of course, is an actual physical injury, an abnormality, or an age-related wearing away of the bone, which may cause or contribute to back pain. These issues may be relatively easy for the medical community to diagnose, but there are many routes to a cure, and we'll talk more about these in Chapter 4. In this chapter, I just want to remind you of our personal mantra: Start with the least invasive treatment and proceed from there. In autumn 2006, the *Journal of the American Medical Association* published a well-designed study that compared patients who had surgery for ruptured discs in their lower backs to those who did not have surgery. Those who had surgery found relief more quickly; however, when the two groups were evaluated 2 years later, the authors noted that the patients who had simply waited eventually improved to the same degree as those who had the surgery. When evaluated 5 to 7 years later, the two groups showed no discernible difference. Although one can't discount the benefit of addressing the pain early through surgery, when you factor in the expense and the possible risk factors, a definite case can be made for simply waiting it out. This means that even if you have one of the classic structural issues that can cause back pain, you don't want to book time with the surgeon just yet. There are many alternatives to surgery, which will be discussed later in the book.

Structural pain can also come from such lifestyle issues as poor posture and too much time sitting with a rounded back at the computer; it can even come from a surprising source, such as years and years of sitting on your wallet. (More about this in Chapter 5.) Iowa researchers examined 15 different studies and found that as little as 20 hours of work at the computer doubles the risk of developing shoulder and arm pain, and over time, shoulder and arm pain often resonate as pain that is felt in the back and neck.

When the muscles and spine are not aligned—often because of bad posture and other lifestyle issues—muscle function, nerve function, and blood supply are compromised. Proper posture and correct use of your muscles make for more effective functioning. Weight lifters understand this concept, and as a result, they are able to lift some impressive weight. When picking something up, most of us hinge at the waist and reach down with our hands. This lifting method compromises our breathing, blood flow, and nerve function. You could never accomplish with this method what a weight lifter could by squatting down first and letting the leg muscles do the real work.

Body form is a vital part of back health and general well-being. Good form permits us to accomplish what we need to without causing injury, and it increases strength and generally optimizes muscular function. Even sedentary acts can be done "better" when proper form is employed. Though sitting at the computer has proven to be a major cause of back pain, you can even do that for prolonged periods if you use proper form. This involves having a good chair, exerting the effort to maintain good posture, and taking regular 5-minute stretching breaks.

Throughout the book, you'll find many suggestions and some specially designed exercises to help you regain proper form so that the pain caused by structural issues will diminish. In the process, you will improve your overall health because your breathing and blood flow will be better able to send nutrients to every part of your body.

Chemical (Nutritional) Causes of Back Pain

"We are what we eat and that can cause back pain" is a statement that always causes patients to raise their eyebrows and look at me quizzically. Their skepticism generally arises because in the Western view of medicine, our bodies are viewed as a nonintegrated collection of separate systems, and the idea that diet could cause back pain is revolutionary. It comes down to the head-scratching question: How could something you eat affect your back?

Because we get such surprised responses when we start asking people about what they eat, there are plenty of days when I think it would be easier to say to a patient, "Yeah, you're right . . . it's that disc that's bothering you. We'll do some adjustments. You should put heat [or ice] on it, and come back next week." Instead, our office is committed to educating our patients on how a chemical or dietary imbalance can contribute to back pain.

Have you ever had a hangover? At some point most people have. And how did you feel? "Nauseous" and "achy all over" are usually among the symptoms. If what you eat or drink has nothing to do with your musculoskeletal system, why do you feel so sick and achy after drinking too much? And what do you do for relief? Usually you take some kind of medication, such as an anti-inflammatory or muscle relaxant. Now you can clearly see the chemical/dietary connection.

Because our bodies are very advanced machines, it makes sense that the quality of the "fuel" we put in it makes a difference. Just as your car functions poorly with dirty oil or conks out without enough gas, your body relies on the excellence of what you put into it.

In Finland, researchers conducted autopsies on people who had died from non-back-related causes but were on record as having suffered from back pain. What they discovered was that people who suffered back pain were more likely to have blocked arteries to the spine than were the comparison group of people who did not have back pain. The average person with back pain was found to have two arteries to the lower back completely blocked and at least one more artery narrowed. This is a notable example of how proper circulation brings nutrients to the spine and removes the cells' waste products. If this isn't happening efficiently, inflammation can result.

Unfortunately, average Americans are not good nutritionists. They'll eat almost anything! It is remarkable how quickly perfectly sane people will take up with the latest fad diet. Shortly after the news media writes about the most recent food-related study, a new diet will have been created to capitalize on the findings. In the early 1990s, everything was low fat, even though some fat is a vital component to health. Then Americans switched to a high-fat, low-carb diet, even though carbohydrates are vital for health.

Now we're swinging toward super-enriched foods, which can also be quite problematic. For example, many breakfast cereals now advertise that they contain 100 percent of our daily requirement of fiber. Although these cereals might be great for you if that's all you ate all day, you don't really need to pack every ounce of fiber into your morning meal. What's wrong with eating healthy foods throughout the day? The same goes regarding the current fad for vitamins and nutritional supplements. Since most of us don't know what we're really eating in the first place, loading up on excess—or even harmful—supplements is not the way to compensate for poor eating habits.

The simple fact is that extremes of anything are not healthy. Too much in the way of simple carbohydrates can lead to diabetes; too much protein can lead to ketoacidosis (a harmful process that breaks down tissues); too much fiber can lead to gas and bloating and digestive issues, all of which can affect arthritis and back pain.

Later in the book we'll discuss dietary changes you can make that will provide proper nutrition to help fight back pain.

Birth Control, Hormonal Treatments, and Back Pain

Both the birth control pill and hormone-replacement therapy (HRT) are possible causes of back pain. Studies have been conducted in Sweden that link oral contraceptives and an increased risk of back problems. Approximately one-quarter of active medical professionals in Sweden now recommend that women who are suffering back pain abandon their use of the birth control pill.

A similar connection has been reported between HRT and back problems. The data were gathered from questionnaires sent to 1,324 women who were 55 to 56 years old and living in Linkoping, Sweden, in 1995; the researchers noted an 85 percent return rate. The study showed a significant association between the use of HRT and lower back pain.

If you're taking oral contraceptives or are using HRT to help you through menopause, consider your level of back pain. If you're truly suffering, perhaps you ought to consider switching off the medications to see if it helps.

Emotional Causes of Back Pain

"God will forgive you but your nervous system will not" is a favorite quote of ours from Hans Selye, a pioneer in the field of stress research. When you experience back pain and your doctor can't find any structural cause, it's reasonable to assume that your pain might be both a symptom and an expression of some distress in your life that generates troubling emotions.

During the last 35 years, researchers have established that the mind–body connection does exist, and it's actually very simple to understand. Scientists now know that stress hormones trigger chronic inflammation and tension in back muscles, tendons, ligaments, and discs. Muscles that contract (read that as tighten up, sometimes too much) need an opportunity to relax, and when you are stressed, the muscles may stay tight, eventually causing great pain. Therefore it is obvious that stress triggers pain—it's not all in your head. When you experience a psychological (mind) imbalance—for example, when you are chronically angry about a problem at work—you also invariably experience a physiological (body) imbalance.

People under stress are sometimes so uncomfortable they think they are having a heart attack. They experience severe chest pains, shortness of breath, and sometimes nausea. When they go to the emergency room, they are told they were having a panic attack, not a heart attack. If emotions can trigger bodily reactions that mimic a heart attack, it is not difficult to understand how negative emotions can set off some very powerful pain mechanisms in your back. The person who is upset about an impending divorce hearing, the one who is anxious about his wedding, and the one who has been caregiver to her parent for several years will all experience stress differently. One may have a migraine, one may have a panic attack, and the other may find herself laid up with back or neck pain. These reactions can all be stress induced.

Sometimes the in-office evaluation leads us to suspect that a patient's pain may have an emotional cause. (Patients would often prefer that we say something like, "Ahhhh . . . I see what the trouble is," or even, "Go home, take two aspirin, and call me in the morning.") These are always the most difficult conversations to have.

"What do you mean I'm stressed?!" is often the response from patients when we mention that a decrease in stress might lead to a decrease in back pain. Although most of us are conditioned to believe that it is a weakness if we have a physical manifestation of how we are feeling, I am here to tell you that's crazy. We all have emotions, and they are going to come out somehow.

Life stresses—and our often negative reactions to them in the form of anger, distress, or fear—are also major triggers of both acute and chronic back pain. Think about it:

- If you're afraid of, or don't enjoy, public speaking or flying, how does your body feel in the hours before a speech or a flight?

- How do you feel when you are waiting for an important phone call, such as news from your parent or child, the outcome of a job interview, or the results of a medical test? How is your breathing? What do you do while waiting? Can you concentrate? Do you have any aches or pains?

When you stop and think about it, you *know* there is a mind–body connection. Every thought and feeling coexists with a set of neurological, hormonal, and even immune-system changes. Your entire biochemistry from moment to moment affects, and is affected by, your thought patterns and emotions. Altered breathing often accompanies these situations and can add to your discomfort. People hold their breath when frightened; they take shallow breaths when nervous—these factors contribute to body pain. When you breathe less deeply, oxygen and nutrients do not circulate around your body at the optimum rate, which results in the formation of a toxic environment. Your muscles tighten up, and you may be in pain until your body has a chance to loosen up.

One Friday, a patient, who is also a friend, called me as he was walking to work. His back was killing him, and he reported that it came "out of the blue." He mentioned that he had a big conference coming up, and he couldn't afford to be sick or have anything be wrong.

I asked him, "Did you do anything differently, strain yourself or sleep on a different mattress?"

The answer was no.

"Did you eat anything differently? Are you feverish? Have your bowel movements been different or are you having any problems while urinating?"

"No."

"Are you feeling stressed?"

"Yes!"

"Bingo," I told him.

Back pain doesn't come from nowhere. If my friend had been eating properly and had no particular reason to worry about a structural issue, then stress was the likely culprit. His muscles were on overdrive because of emotional strain. Some people get headaches, other people's jaws clamp up; still others feel the tightness in their backs.

We talked for a few more minutes about the upcoming conference he was worried about, and we discussed his options: Could he knock off work early that day (no), go for a massage Saturday morning (another no), or at least sleep a little extra Friday night (yes)?

When I called him the following Saturday, his back pain was gone. He said that simply figuring out that it was stress allowed him to calm down a bit.

One of my favorite success stories is my patient Risa, who comes in every few months whenever her hip starts to hurt. She's told me that when she begins to notice muscle tension as a result of stress, she simply focuses on what is stressing her out. Within 10 minutes the pain usually goes away.

Why the Three-Tiered Approach Works

As you continue reading this book, you'll come to better understand that what you eat or how you feel can provoke back pain that is every bit as debilitating as pain from whiplash, arthritis, and other physical causes. When we work with our patients, the effectiveness of our diagnoses and remedies prove that this is true. But this is not to say that the diagnostics of back pain are easy.

For one thing, the symptoms may arise from more than one source. After all, how many people eat really healthfully when they are stressed out? The interaction of these influences can make a diagnosis very complex.

Can pain come solely from a structural issue? Absolutely, but that doesn't always call for surgery. Recently I saw a patient who entered the office complaining of neck and shoulder pain that has bothered her consistently for the past 3 years. Though she had seen other chiropractors and physical therapists, she had complained to me that nothing had ever seemed to help for any prolonged period of time.

During the initial examination, it became pretty evident that even though the symptoms were located in her neck and shoulders, her problem was rooted in something much deeper than just those locations. By taking a postural evaluation of her, I noticed that one shoulder was higher than the other, one hip was considerably higher than the other, and one leg was longer than the other. From this evaluation, I knew that her shoulder and neck symptoms were secondary and that her postural imbalance was the primary cause of her problems. My suspicion was that the other professionals had worked on only her neck and shoulders. We worked out a plan involving stretches and exercises as well as chiropractic corrections. These were designed to correct her postural imbalance, and once her alignment was better, we had less to do to reduce the tightness that had settled in her neck and shoulders.

Diagnoses are all the more complicated because the body has a natural order. The primary cause of the problem needs to be corrected before you can have a long-term effect on what, in many cases, are the more bothersome secondary symptoms. This may mean sacrificing the short-term feel-good type of treatment for the fix that will work over the long term. For example, had I focused on only the neck and shoulder issues of my recent patient, her pain would have continued.

The message to you is to be a patient patient. If your first attempt doesn't work, stay focused on other possibilities. The amazing thing about taking care of the primary factors first is the number of secondary symptoms that disappear soon after.

Why Don't You Listen?

"Why don't you listen?" was a frequent question I heard from my mother when I was growing up. As annoyed as I was when she would ask it, there was generally some life lesson I had missed or not paid attention to, and she was pointing this out to me.

Today this question is one that everyone should ask themselves when it comes to back pain: Why don't you listen? The pain you are feeling is your body screaming for attention. When someone comes into the office after weeks or months of suffering and tells me that they had hoped the pain would just go away but mostly it just gets worse, it upsets me. Would you ignore a warning light on your car or the beep of a smoke detector? Of course not! But why do we seem so willing to do so when it comes to our health? If a pet gets ill, most owners immediately take the pet to the vet. Yet when it comes to their own health, people will wait days, weeks, and months, thinking their pain will go away. Sometimes they turn to an over-the-counter remedy, which they end up taking for weeks on end. It makes me crazy!

Mario is an active, physically fit guy in his mid-40s, who plays tennis four times a week on a very intense and competitive level. During a recent office visit he was quite uncomfortable, complaining of knee, back, and neck pain both before and after he exercised. Before he came to me he had begun popping a couple of over-the-counter painkillers before each workout. He told me: "It made a big difference. It didn't hurt as much when I played."

I cannot begin to tell you how often I hear that a patient takes a pain reliever before he or she starts to exercise. Taking acetaminophen or ibuprofen a couple times a year for a headache or a sprained ankle can be helpful; however, the frequency with which people are taking these drugs is downright harmful and dangerous. These medications can lead to internal bleeding, and every year anti-inflammatory drugs cause the hospitalization of approximately 70,000 people for perforated ulcers or severe gastrointestinal bleeding. If we discount the actual injury that can come from taking too much of these pain relievers or by taking them too often, then we are left with the point I was making earlier. By muffling the sound of what your body is telling you, you are running the risk of sustaining a major injury. If your body feels abnormally sore and achy or you experience pain from exercise, it is your body's attempt to tell you that something is wrong. This is your defense mechanism that allows you to avoid activities that do you harm.

If some part of your body hurts, listen. If you take care of it now, before long you'll be back on the tennis courts, the ball field, or the machines at the gym— pain-free.

Back Pain Is Often a Good Thing

Back pain could be the greatest thing that ever happened to you. You don't want to miss this opportunity to listen and learn from the message that back pain can bring. You can use this opportunity to change your life forever, or you can ignore the message and continue an unhealthy lifestyle.

The time has come to start paying attention to the hints your body gives you. These hints come in the form of tension, tightness, weakness, and pain. You should not ignore these signs and hope they will go away. The preventive approach is always best. When you listen to your body, the result is less pain and greater vitality and flexibility, the hallmarks of true health.

Most of us do not even realize how poorly we feel because we are so used to feeling subpar. But remember: It is not normal to be sore after playing a round of golf. Nor is it normal to wake up stiff and achy just because you are 60 years old. Stop accepting such a low level of function for your back, and don't believe all the hype that tells you that your spine will deteriorate as you age. I hope this book provides you with a better understanding and approach to optimal spinal and back health.

The next chapter puts you on the road to self-diagnosis.

Assessing Your Situation

I would never presume to tell my accountant how to fill in the fine points on my tax return, nor would I ever think of giving my dentist instructions on how to fill my tooth, but it is my responsibility with both of these experts to provide them with as much helpful information as I can. To do the best job he can for me, my accountant needs complete documentation of all my business expenses, carefully organized—not in a shoe box I dump on his desk. My dentist needs guidance on what in my mouth is bothering me, such as whether I have a tooth that's sensitive to cold, a tooth that actually hurts, or a jaw that aches. If I provide these professionals with reliable information, they will be best prepared to help me.

You have this same responsibility of accurate reporting on your overall health picture, but here it gets complicated. Most of us have just one dentist, but we all have, or know of, multiple medical doctors. While being able to consult a dermatologist for skin problems and see a podiatrist for bunions is helpful in solving site-specific, clear issues, we encounter problems when the illness or the cause of the pain is more general or less well defined. Who does one consult about a headache, back pain, arthritis, or stomach ills? There are many options, and diagnoses are problematic because each professional knows his or her own field best. What's more, who you see determines what type of treatment you get: If you are complaining of lower back pain and you start with a primary care doctor, she may do some tests and reach for the prescription pad to give you anti-inflammatories. If you see a chiropractor, he'll provide manipulations. If you ask your physical therapist, she will provide exercises for strength and stretching. And if you make the mistake of going to a surgeon too soon, you may be undergoing surgery earlier than necessary. (And, unfortunately, our current healthcare model creates competition among the specialties.) And yet any one of these people may hold the key to fixing what ails you. How can you possibly know where to turn?

And that's the purpose of this chapter. In our practice, we've established a series of questions that we use to help pinpoint the source of the trouble. The questions are basic enough that you can run through them on your own and, in doing so, begin to better understand the source of your back pain. Once you understand that, you'll know whether you need a medical professional and, if so, what specialty you need to pursue. For example, if the questions point to a dietary cause of your back pain, you can start by adjusting your diet or by visiting a nutritionist.

But first we want to introduce you to some basic rules we follow in any type of back pain diagnosis. Above all, you want to be safe, and these rules will remind you of the importance of proceeding methodically and getting help when necessary.

The Nine Rules of Back Pain Diagnosis

Rule 1: Make sure you are not dealing with anything more serious than back pain.

On occasion, back pain can be a sign of something more serious (an infection, a tumor, or cancer), but this is *not* usually the case. Check with your primary care physician if you have any of the following symptoms:

- The back pain wakes you up at night.
- You have bladder or bowel problems that began about the same time as the back pain.
- You have a fever, even a low-grade one.

A primary care doctor will perform a physical examination and order blood work and a urinalysis. Some may order an X-ray, a test we find to be much more helpful than the more modern MRI. X-rays allow the doctor to see the bone structure as well as any spinal wear and tear caused by lifestyle issues or poor posture. An X-ray will also reveal growths or signs of infection. (I recently found a benign tumor on a patient's spine that would have turned malignant had it not been for the early detection via X-ray studies.)

While most primary care doctors have not received specialized training in managing back pain, they are certainly prepared to rule out worrisome issues. Just remember that they may not be your last stop when looking for a solution to back pain. There are many other types of professionals who are well prepared to focus on the specific cause of your back pain.

Rule 2: The only thing random in the body is trauma.

For the most part, back pain is a lot more predictable than people think. As we have noted, the only time pain stems from a "random" source is when someone has fallen, been in a car accident, or otherwise experienced bodily trauma. All other types of back pain have built up gradually over time. Bending over to pick up something does not cause back pain on its own; you've likely been doing small bits of damage over time. Even minor violations of the natural laws of back health (refer to Chapter 1) can result in severe pain if they compound themselves over time.

Rule 3: If you ask the wrong questions, you will get the wrong answers.

The main reason we have so much back pain is because patients and health professionals are asking the wrong questions. Up until now, the standard assessment questions have addressed only the possible structural causes of back pain. These wrong questions lead to wrong answers, which lead to invasive treatments and little to no prospect of helping you.

Rule 4: Start with the least invasive diagnosis and treatment methods, and proceed to the more invasive ones only if absolutely necessary.

Doctors learn early on *primum non nocere*, "First, do no harm." As you'll read in this book, there are some lifestyle changes that may help your back pain. If you can change your lifestyle and make your pain go away, why would you start taking medicines or proceed with surgery? Numerous peer-reviewed journals estimate that there are 100,000 deaths a year and a million people severely injured because of adverse reactions to prescription drugs. (Adverse drug interactions kill more people than do automobile and airplane accidents combined.) Although there are times when medication and/or surgery are the only cures, it is important to remember these options are not risk-free, so it is important to go from least invasive to more invasive.

I once heard someone say, "To the hammer, the world looks like a nail," and this can certainly be true when it comes to the various forms of medicine. Doctors are most comfortable with the solutions that they have been trained to use. Studies verify this: If back pain patients see an orthopedic surgeon before consulting with other healthcare providers, there is an increased likelihood that they will undergo surgery. This isn't to condemn orthopedic surgeons—it would be the same with other professionals as well. We are all best at what we know.

If you start with a less-invasive treatment method and fail to get results, you can always move on to a different specialty. Unfortunately, it is very difficult to go the other way.

Rule 5: Everyone is different.

Every case is unique. Even if two people have the exact same symptoms, they may need to be treated in two totally separate and distinct ways. Because each person may have different contributing factors, the best approach is to apply the three-tiered assessment to get to the root of each person's problem.

Rule 6: There is no one answer; a variety of professions and approaches may be beneficial.

This book is certainly not intended to put any specialist out of business. Depending on what is determined to be the cause of the pain, a patient may benefit from physical therapy, acupuncture, chiropractic work, nutritional guidance, psychological help, and even surgery.

Unfortunately, many specialists don't agree; and because they don't believe in a coordinated effort, they have made treating back pain a competitive sport, with the patient definitely being the loser. For example, if you see a neurologist for head and neck pain, she may not believe in chiropractic care. As a result, even if she fails to treat you effectively, she may not refer you on to see if you can get relief elsewhere. By dismissing certain types of care (chiropractic, acupuncture, and stress relief are usually low on the list for referrals from other professionals), doctors reduce your options for finding a solution.

Different professions should not be viewed as separate, competing entities; they each have their specialty, and a different approach may be just what you need. By using the three-tiered assessment outlined later in this chapter, you will be sure that you are seeing the right practitioner to alleviate your back problem.

Rule 7: Do one thing at a time.

No matter how bad your pain, your search for a solution needs to be methodical. A scattershot, try-everything approach will not prove instructive. Because pain can recur, it's important to learn as much as you can about the underlying cause.

> A woman named Wendy arrived in our offices saying that she had been suf-
> fering from severe migraine headaches that came almost daily for the past 3
> years. She was at her wit's end and was desperate for a solution. As we ex-
> plored her situation, she mentioned that she was seeing a neurologist, taking
> numerous medications, starting Botox treatments (which can sometimes be
> helpful in headache pain relief), and considering acupuncture. Although
> desperation had made her frantic for a solution, I explained to her that the
> only way to find a solution was to slow down and try one thing at a time.

If you take a scattershot approach, you won't be able to unravel what is helpful and what isn't. Trying too many things at the same time may actually make the situation worse. When it comes to back pain, too many cooks can spoil the broth.

Rule 8: Be a patient patient; just don't be too patient.

In our practice, we believe in the 6-week rule. If you are not significantly better within 6 weeks, something is not right. Why 6 weeks? Six weeks provides enough opportunity for a doctor's recommendations to work. If the suggested remedy is not working, the patient has not wasted much time on a treatment.

However, after 6 weeks with little or no results, it is time to move on and look for another solution.

Another mistake patients sometimes make is not trying something for long enough. For a couple of weeks they'll do the set of exercises recommended by the physical therapist, and then they'll give up. "It didn't help," they'll tell us. Well, of course it didn't help! Who ever accomplished a life change after 10 to 14 days of some basic exercises? Although you don't want to get into a treatment rut, you do want to give any therapy a full try. Six weeks is a good general time frame to figure out whether something is working.

Not all patients are good patients; if people don't do the exercises or change their eating habits or take the medication as prescribed, they probably aren't going to get better. What's more, the disobedient patient makes life much more complicated for himself. When patients don't give a full effort to seeing if something works, it's very difficult to help these people solve their problems.

I also advise people, "Don't give up your bitching rights. You have to follow the plan for 6 weeks or so. If you do so and fail to get results, then you have the right to bitch."

Rule 9: Your immune system plays a big part in keeping you pain-free.

Stay healthy. If you should encounter back pain, a good immune system will make you more resilient. A person who drinks a lot of coffee, eats junk food, and sits on a lot of airplanes is more likely to suffer from back pain than the person in my waiting room who is relaxed and eats healthily. The person who enjoys good health can sleep on a poor mattress now and then, lift something improperly, or even twist the wrong way during exercise. While this person may have a bad day or two from the immediate trauma, chances are excellent that he or she will rebound quickly.

What a Doctor Should Ask You

While it would be nice if each and every reader could come to our offices for a diagnosis, I know that's not possible. Instead, we've created a diagnostic system you can use on your own. By pursuing the leads you get from asking yourself the questions listed in the following sections, you may be able to make some lifestyle corrections that will start the healing process. Or the answers may show you which professional can help you in your pursuit of pain relief. This will save you time in your search for a cure.

As you know, we believe the key to freeing you from back problems is getting to an accurately diagnosed cause. Our relatively simple assessment tool can help you get there.

There are three parts to the assessment: questions pertaining to the structural, chemical, and emotional realms. Be sure to go through the complete assessment. Most of the time back pain is a combination of the three.

Your Personal Back Health Assessment

Is It Structural?
Remember here that the only thing random in the body is trauma. If you were fine and fell off your bike, then any pain you are suffering probably came about because you fell off your bike—that's random. Otherwise, pain due to a structural cause is *not* random, and it doesn't occur because you suddenly bent wrong and your back went out. This type of structural pain tends to be caused by a buildup of bad habits (sitting slumped over at the computer or watching TV with your neck bent forward) or a prolonged misuse of your body, which can develop in someone with bad posture. Consider the following questions:

- ❏ Did you recently exercise differently?

- ❏ Did you recently lift anything heavier than normal?

- ❏ Have you done a lot of sit-ups or crunches?

- ❏ Do you sit at a computer for long periods at a time?

- ❏ Have you been traveling a lot?

- ❏ Were you doing different types of work, such as shoveling snow or raking leaves?

❑   Were you bent over in an unusual posture for a long period of time?

❑   Were you wearing different shoes?

If you answered yes to one or more of these questions, make a note of which one(s). One yes answer does not give you a diagnosis!

Is It Chemical?

What you eat—whether it's too much coffee, too many sweets, or a host of other edibles that are unique to you (and further explored in Chapters 7 to 9)—can keep your digestive system "agitated," and this can result in chemically induced back pain. With dietary issues, we are looking for either changes in the chemical system or repetitive patterns that can result in back pain.

❑   Have you been constipated recently?

❑   Have you had diarrhea recently?

❑   Has your stomach been bothering you?

❑   Have you had an increase in gas?

❑   Have you eaten any types of food that you don't normally consume?

❑   Do you repetitively eat the same foods?

❑   Have you eaten spicy foods recently?

❑   Have you recently had a stomach virus?

❑   Have you been on any new medications?

❑   Have you changed your diet?

❑   Have you changed your vitamin regimen?

❑   Have you increased your fiber intake?

❑   Have you recently started to drink something different?

❑   Did you recently have abnormal amounts of alcohol?

❑   Do you drink a good deal of coffee or soda?

❑   Do you eat foods that are high in sugar?

❑   Do you use an artificial sweetener? If so, which one?

❑   Did you just begin your menstrual period?

❑   Has your hormonal system undergone any recent changes
     (menopause, change in birth control, missed menstrual period,
     etc.)?

*If you answered yes to one or more of these questions, make a note of which
one(s). Then be sure to go through the rest of the questions.*

Is It Emotional?

Stress causes tight muscles, and tight muscles can cause serious pain. Although
people are often reluctant to admit to an emotional cause for back pain, it is very
important to be open-minded about this, as we find that stress is a major contributor to back pain. (You'll read more about this later in the book.)

❑   How would you describe your current stress level?

❑   Has any area of your life been more stressful recently?

❑   Are you under particular stress at work?

❑   Are you getting along with your fellow employees?

❑   Do you feel better during the weekend as opposed to the week?

❑   Has there recently been a change in your relationships with your fam-
     ily members and friends?

❑   Has a close family member or friend recently undergone an illness or a
     death?

❑   Have you recently had any financial problems?

❑   Are you feeling fulfilled in your career?

❑   Did you recently have to do something that you didn't want to do?

❑   Do you frequently feel anxious?

❑   Where do you seem to carry your stress? Most people register stress
     in the upper half of their bodies. Are you someone who suffers from

headaches, tight neck, shoulder tension, or lower back pain? Even an upset stomach can develop from an emotional cause.

❑   Are you trying to get pregnant and having difficulty doing so?

❑   Are you having difficulty sleeping?

❑   Are you feeling stressed out and worried because of the pain you are suffering?

❑   Is anything else in your life happening that makes you feel stressed?

You may be surprised at how many yes responses you have here. Our lives aren't simple! But because 85 percent of people suffer back pain at some point in their lives, it isn't surprising to have a good number of positive responses in this realm.

When You Hear Hoofbeats, Think Horses

"When you hear hoofbeats, think horses, not zebras" is a humorous way of reminding young medical professionals to explore the obvious before the esoteric. The same reminder applies to the diagnostic exercise in this book. Take a look at the notes you've made based on the preceding questions. You have to play the percentages. If you've been under a great deal of stress lately and have noted yes to many of the questions in the emotional section, then turn to Part IV and start out with de-stressing as a form of pain relief. If you have been traveling a lot or have been on a work deadline, crunched up at your computer, then turn first to Part II, which addresses structural issues.

If You Need a Professional Consultation

Most people who read this book will recognize their symptoms rather quickly. When you think about it, you'll realize that the fifth cup of coffee you have each day may be causing part of your problem, or you'll see that the fact that you are going through a divorce is likely a major cause of your back pain. Or you'll begin to give more thought to your posture. If you identify one of these issues as being more likely to be causing your problem, then you'll be able to use the recommendations presented later in the book to bring about a solution to your problem.

However, you may feel stuck and want to turn to someone for help. I don't blame you for feeling confused—there are many options, so here are some guidelines for finding a professional who might be helpful in your circumstances.

First, because back pain often results from a group of imbalances, the ideal first-stop professional is one who is willing to take a holistic, whole-body approach to back pain. As discussed, you want to start with the least invasive types of solutions, moving on only as needed. A surgeon should never be the first person you see if you are suffering from back pain.

Remember that there are all types of professionals who are wonderful diagnosticians (in many fields) but who have no patience or who have a terrible bedside manner. You want someone who will listen to you well enough that he or she really hears what you are saying. It makes all the difference. Generally, the best way to find these folks is through word of mouth. Ask friends, relatives, and coworkers about their experiences. What was the nature of their back problem? What did their healthcare professional recommend? Has the problem been solved? If so, how long did it take?

And no matter what type of professional you visit, don't necessarily expect him or her to get it right immediately. Most people aren't very good at describing their pain—it's difficult to find the right words, and it's difficult to provide all the right puzzle pieces for the professional on a first visit. Look for someone you like, and remember that he or she should be making new decisions based on your feedback after the first visit or two. If the healthcare provider is a "my way or the highway" type, look for someone else.

If the Problem Is Structural

If your primary issue seems to be structural, then you want to see a professional who specializes in the structure of the spine. Personally, I would start with a chiropractor. Chiropractors are trained in natural treatments of the spine that affect the bones as well as the muscles.

An ideal team for a structural issue may involve a chiropractor, a physical therapist, and a massage therapist. (We use this team approach in our offices.)

Physical therapists are specialists in muscle rehabilitation and can provide great results in treating muscle-related back pain. Massage therapists undergo 2 to 3 years of training in manual ways to loosen the musculature that, when tight, can cause pain.

For some symptoms (numbness or tingling, for example), I would consult an orthopedist early on. He or she can then take a very thorough look at your spine. An orthopedist can also prescribe muscle relaxants and anti-inflammatory medications, which can be very helpful if used for limited periods. After this immediate relief, however, you will probably need a chiropractor or physical therapist to help with a long-term fix.

If the Problem Is Chemical

If you determine that your problem is dietary, start with the anti-back-pain diet provided in this book. Try it for 3 or 4 weeks before consulting a professional. Though the 6-week rule is recommended to give most other types of treatment a chance, our bodies are more responsive to chemical changes. If you make changes that affect your body chemistry positively (or negatively), you'll see the effects in as little as 3 weeks.

During that time, start a food diary, recording what you eat and drink every day for 7 days. Based on the information in Part III, you may clearly see where you have gone wrong. If not, a food diary will be very helpful to any professional you consult.

If you try the anti-back-pain diet for 3 weeks, but you are still having pain, then visit a primary care doctor or gastroenterologist to see if there are any underlying illnesses that might be causing your chemical imbalance. If the tests are all negative, then visit a nutritionist who will be able to examine your particular situation and get you on the road to recovery. Ask around for someone who is smart, flexible, and good at coming up with new ideas. Some nutritionists have very specific specialties (eating disorders or diabetes, for example), and these professionals may offer the type of help you need.

If the Problem Is Emotional

Many of our patients achieve relief just by coming to the realization that stress is causing their pain. If so, you may feel better already. If not, spend some time evaluating the stress in your life and examining how you deal with it. Part IV offers advice on methods that can help counter emotion-related back pain.

If you are still experiencing pain, consider consulting a mental health professional. Someone in this type of profession—therapist, social worker, psychologist, or psychiatrist—is trained to help you identify the cause of your emotional troubles and then help you deal with your problems.

It's Not Rocket Science, But . . .

Annette is a very active and healthy woman in her early 60s. She practices yoga and eats healthily. But because she was in a car accident a couple of years ago, Annette sees me about 10 times a year for chiropractic treatments.

Recently, Annette complained of lower back pain for the first time. She'd learned enough from our sessions that she immediately thought, "What have I been doing differently?" She decided that her back pain must have come from sleeping on a soft bed at a hotel, and she reported to me that she was going to be more careful about the types of beds that she slept on. Although her reasoning made a certain amount of sense, I knew Annette was too strong, too healthy, and too fit to be suffering from a few nights on a soft bed, so we talked for a bit about what else might be contributing to her back pain.

When we went through some questions together (Have you eaten differently? Has your stomach been upset? Have you been particularly stressed recently?), we determined that her back pain came on from tension due to work stress. Her company was going through a difficult period, her workload had increased but her pay had been cut, and many good friends she had worked with for years had just been laid off. Her muscles went into spasm because she was uptight and stressed because of work.

Not only was she thrilled when I told her she was not deteriorating and that she was too healthy to get back pain from a couple of bad nights, but she realized what was at the root of her pain, and that put her back on the road to living pain-free. (Worrying about the why of pain simply leads to even more pain because you become tense from it.)

Because I knew that Annette had excellent structural and muscle balance, and because I knew that she was careful with her diet, it was easy for me to deduce that the cause of her additional pain was emotional.

Your goal is to get to the point where you understand yourself so well that you, too, know what direction to explore when you are in pain.

PART TWO

The Head Bone's Connected to the Neck Bone: The Structural Causes of Back Pain

CHAPTER 4

Look at the Big Picture
to Find the Remedy

For 3½ years, Mike had been suffering from debilitating back pain, which led him to pursue multiple avenues in search of a solution. He had X-rays, MRI studies, and CT scans by request of his doctors. He tried acupuncture, traditional chiropractic adjustments, massage, and a variety of exercise routines in an effort to relieve the pain. Nothing worked.

When I met Mike, he was quite discouraged and admitted that his doctors had begun to indicate that his problem might be psychosomatic—something with which Mike was having trouble coming to terms because to him the pain didn't feel like something that was all in his head.

"I think they are missing something, Dr. Sinett," Mike told me.

After I took a history of his health and back pain, I conducted a full head-to-toe examination, as I always do with any new patient. In the process, I noted that Mike's legs were markedly uneven, throwing his pelvis out of alignment. As I continued to evaluate the possible cause of this distortion, I took a quick glance at Mike's shoes, which were sitting to one side in the examining room. Based on an evaluation of his physical condition—and his shoes—I noted that Mike had a condition known as pronation, a degeneration of the arches of his feet, which was causing his body to be out of alignment. I had my answer to Mike's back pain.

I conducted several adjustments to provide Mike with some immediate relief, and I sent him to be fit with customized orthotic insoles that he now wears in all of his shoes. (Such shoe inserts are custom-made to correct a person's individual problem and can be slipped in and out of multiple pairs of shoes.) Mike came for a few more visits, but within 6 weeks, our basic work was done. He sent me the following note: "I am thrilled to report that I am pain-free and feeling 10 years younger. It is amazing what pain does to one's body, mind, and spirit. I did not realize how much it impacted my energy and general mood."

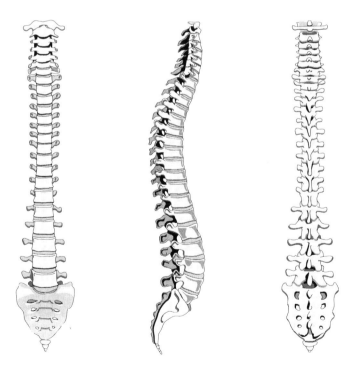

Figure 1. The anatomy of the spine.

Does the fact that Mike's feet were giving him a back ache surprise you? It does most people, particularly those who come to us with pain in one area of the body and learn that the cause of the pain stems from something else entirely.

We'll explore this issue later in the chapter, but first it's important that you have a better understanding of the body's structure.

The Anatomy of the Spine

The spine is a dynamic structure designed for both strength and flexibility. It has two major functions:

- **TO KEEP US UPRIGHT.** Without it, we might be wormlike in our movements.

- **TO PROTECT THE SPINAL CORD.** The spinal cord houses "operation body control" for all of us. The brain's messages travel to our outlying nerves via this vital column, which is a fundamental component of our body's regulation system.

The spine structure is quite complex. The column itself consists of 33 bones, called *vertebrae*. Twenty-four of these vertebrae are mobile and give the body and spine its flexibility:

- Seven vertebrae in the neck, which are designed for movement.
- Twelve vertebrae in the mid-back, which connect to the rib cage.
- Five vertebrae in the lower back, which are designed to handle the weight and stress of the body.

An additional 9 vertebrae are at the end of the spine—the sacrum, your tailbone—and are fixed. They are vital for stability.

The vertebrae—both mobile and immobile—are linked, and they are connected by joints called *facets*. These facets are separated by *discs*, which are jelly-like in substance. The discs provide both stability and cushioning to the overall spine. (If the bones of the spine had no cushioning, each step we took would be quite jarring.)

Muscles and ligaments—lots of them—are attached to the vertebrae. Each of these muscles performs certain actions that play an integrated role in overall function. Imbalance in any one of these muscles can throw off the intricate balance of the spine. Continued imbalance results in a decrease in function and, often, pain.

Referred Pain

People—doctors included—feel that wherever the pain is located is also the location of the problem. Many professionals divide a back examination into parts, such as lower back, mid-back, and upper back. Then the doctor examines and treats the area in which the patient is experiencing the pain. A person suffering from lower back pain will receive orthopedic and neurological tests and perhaps X-ray or MRI studies. The medical professional will then probably recommend that the patient receive some physiotherapy or exercises for the lower back. This local approach is misguided, analogous to someone lost in the forest who looks at the trees only within a few feet of where he or she is. By looking only regionally, we are missing the overall picture when treating back pain.

Unfortunately, even insurance companies subscribe to this theory. Many will pay for examinations or tests that pertain only to the exact area of the body about which the patient is complaining. Everything else will be denied based on what they consider medical necessity—a true pity, because this philosophy is so wrong.

We are here to tell you that we have learned that an injury or an imbalance in one place can trigger pain and discomfort someplace else entirely. In fact, frequently where the pain is, the problem is not.

Remember that song "Dem Bones," which we all learned in kindergarten? *The head bone's connected to the neck bone . . .* and so on.

We have seen thousands of cases in which the patient comes in complaining of lower back pain, yet the problem is actually coming from their feet or their neck or their hips. Or the person with shoulder pain may actually be suffering from a problem with their neck or mid-back. People who break their ankles frequently develop back pain. Can you guess why? Because when they hobble around favoring the injured foot, it throws everything else out of whack, causing pain.

A Closed Kinetic Chain

If you visualize your spine as a shoelace, it will provide you with a very good picture of what I'm going to describe to you. Take that shoelace and see what happens if you staple one end of the lace to a piece of paper (representing the rest of your body) and let the other end of the shoelace hang down from the edge. Now start twisting the loose end of the shoelace. If you twist long enough, you'll find that the entire shoelace—as well as the piece of paper that represents your body—gets all twisted.

So if you think of the shoelace as a stand-in for your spine, you begin to understand why we have long believed that what happens in one location in your spine most definitely affects the rest of your back. The spine is completely integrated; every part relates to your entire body.

Always remember that we are a synchronous integrated machine. If you view your body as consisting of multiple separate and distinct parts, the likelihood of you ridding yourself of back pain forever is nearly impossible.

When we conduct a chiropractic examination, we consider the body as a whole, and we check for some things that might surprise you.

Looking for the Cause of Pain

When a detective first comes upon a crime scene, he or she rules out no one as a suspect—mother, brother, sister, lover: Anyone and everyone is under suspicion until the crime is solved. We approach each patient as a detective works a crime. We start with a global approach, and as we work, we take an ever-narrower focus on the cause of the back problem.

When it comes to hunting down the cause of pain, my father taught me the importance of considering a patient's whole body. A complete examination—head to toe no matter what the complaint—leads to some puzzled looks when we are examining a patient's neck even though he or she has arrived concerned about lower back pain, but it is an integral part of helping us understand how to make people feel better.

Proper Alignment Head to Toe

Good chiropractors do a complete examination, regardless of the patient's complaint. We begin our look at a patient's ear levels, which should appear even from right to left. If a patient has one ear higher or lower than the other, we know that he or she has a condition called *head tilt*. An uneven head tilt can create discomfort in the upper neck area as a result of this muscular imbalance.

We also look at the patient's jaw. Does the patient have a symmetrical jaw? If not, the patient's likelihood of suffering from temporomandibular joint (TMJ) symptoms is greatly increased. Such symptoms can come from a clenching of the jaw, which can easily be the cause of severe headaches and neck, jaw, and even ear pain.

How is the curve of the neck? If a patient appears to carry his or her head too far forward, the muscles have difficulty supporting it.

Moving down the spine, we evaluate shoulder heights. The shoulders should be evenly balanced from left to right. If one shoulder appears higher than the other, it is a clue that the patient could be suffering from some shoulder and neck pain due to the imbalance. It is also important to see if one shoulder is rotated forward in relation to the other. If so, this is a clue that mid-back pain is not too far behind. A shoulder that is rotated forward puts a lot of pressure on the shoulder-blade area of the back. A shoulder imbalance could be coming from the hips or neck as well as from the shoulders themselves. There are many nerves that exit the neck, pass through the shoulder area, and supply the elbows and hands. You might be surprised to learn that imbalanced shoulder heights can cause a patient to suffer carpal tunnel or forearm and wrist pain.

We then look at how a patient's arms hang. Are they symmetrical? If the hands are rotated inward or excessively outward, this would indicate a shoulder imbalance.

As we continue through our postural checklist, we look at the pelvis and umbilical region. Are the hips even, and is the pelvis centered? When the hips are at different heights or are rotated, the patient may experience a multitude of symptoms, including lower back pain. Next, we evaluate the knees. Are they bowed? Are they symmetrical? Knee positioning is very important and indicates whether the body is properly aligned while standing.

Finally, we look at a patient's feet for imbalances, for the nature of the arches, and for any foot or toe issues that may impede normal body biomechanics. (More about this later in the chapter.)

When someone suffers from one or more of these imbalances, does it mean that he or she will be in pain? No! Does it dramatically increase the chance that that person will be in pain? Yes! Poor posture puts pressure in areas that were not meant to handle it. The result is a decrease in range of motion and the overall elasticity of the body. These imbalances also greatly increase the chance of getting hurt during exercise or some other type of exertion.

When we do a structural examination, the actual symptoms are secondary to getting the body in structural alignment. Remember that everything is related. After proper alignment is achieved, people are amazed by how many other symptoms go away. After the basic structural examination, there are some other alignment issues and body usage issues that we always check for.

It Starts with a Strong Base: The Pelvis

When I talk to patients, I describe the pelvis—the lowest portion of the spine— as the foundation of their house. Their head, neck, and shoulders all rely on that base remaining strong.

If a person's pelvis is not aligned properly, it can easily affect the hips and the entire lower extremities, including the knees and legs. During the initial examination I will always look for balance within the pelvis. This assessment is easily accomplished by placing one's hands on each side of a person's hips. Ideally the examiner's hands should line up perfectly, but this frequently is not the case. The extent and degree to which a person's pelvis is off balance can easily be measured by taking an X-ray of the lower back. The larger the differential between each side of the pelvis, the greater the chances are that the patient is suffering from back pain because of this. (Patients sometimes mention that their tailor has noted that one pant leg needs to be longer than the other because of a physical discrepancy.) Rather than it being an anatomical problem (and perhaps something you were born with), it is usually a postural one, meaning it is something that has developed throughout your lifetime. This type of imbalance can come from something as simple as sitting on a wallet that is in your back pocket all day. (See Chapter 5 for additional lifestyle habits that can cause back pain.)

Consider the Way You Walk

Another important element of a good chiropractic examination is *gait analysis*—how the patient walks. We are always on the move, and how we walk is as important as how we sit. Although attention is often given to choosing a proper chair, it is equally important for patients to work at good posture and improving their gait.

Though humans use only two of their four limbs to walk, the rest of the body is very much in motion. If we take a step forward with our right foot, our right arm will swing backward, and the left side moves in opposition. During this seemingly simple process, all of our muscles must fire in a synchronous manner, with some muscles tightening while their counterparts relax. When the front main leg muscle (called the quadriceps) contracts, the back of the leg muscle (the hamstring) relaxes. This is what allows us to move forward. If all of the muscles contracted at the same time, we would be stuck in one position with a giant spasm. If this intricate walking mechanism is thrown off balance, people can literally walk themselves into back pain.

The Three Phases of Proper Walking

- **PHASE 1: THE HEEL STRIKE.** The point when your heel first makes contact with the ground.

- **PHASE 2: FLAT FOOT.** When the rest of your foot hits the ground.

- **PHASE 3: PUSH OFF OR TOE OFF.** When your big toe and then the rest of your toes push you off the ground, propelling you forward.

Remember that walking is a full-body occupation—both arms and legs are in motion, which is one of the reasons it's so good for your health. As mentioned, when you step with the right leg forward, your left arm swings forward at the same time. This twist of your arm creates momentum in your mid-back to propel you forward in an efficient manner.

Once in a while, walk more slowly than usual and focus on both your posture and your form. Learning the proper way to walk takes time like any other skill. Focus on two things: the synchronization of your arms and legs, and the proper striking and toeing off of your feet.

The Importance of the Feet

As evidenced by Mike's situation described at the beginning of this chapter, a good number of structural back problems often stem from the feet.

The foot has three arches. When properly maintained with decent shoes and proper gait, these arches lift the weight evenly and, in doing so, provide excellent support. Many people stand unevenly, and certain parts of the foot's sole are not carrying their end of the bargain, which can result in back pain. Other parts of the feet pick up the slack, but the result is an imbalance that reverberates through the spine—top to bottom. This cumulative, repetitive imbalance is generally a result of a postural imbalance that lies within the feet.

Although I always check out the foot itself, a quick glance at the patient's shoes will reveal a lot. (If you are frequently taking your shoes to the shoemaker to correct an uneven amount of wear on your shoes, then you know what I mean.) Both shoes should wear down the same way at the same rate. If this does not occur, you can safely assume that your feet are not in balance, and back pain is not too far behind.

The patient's choice of shoe style can also make a big difference in back health and back pain. I see this every day in my office. Patients frequently arrive in great-looking shoes that are not the healthiest of choices. The heels are too high or the toes are too pointy or the shoes have been made with no thought to stability and thus the wearer risks a sprain or break. Summertime is a particular problem when people—both men and women—start wearing flip-flops, open shoes, sandals, and loafers. These shoes provide little support, and in the case of some sandals and flip-flops, your muscles have to contort just to keep the shoe on your foot. (See the next chapter for advice on proper footwear.)

The Forward Head Tilt

How many times have you observed someone reading a newspaper with her head thrust forward? Or think about the posture of the last person who drove you somewhere—did he drive with his head jutting forward? (Do you recognize yourself when thinking about this posture?) Many of the patients I see suffer from neck pain brought on by poor postural habits. It seems that modern life has given us lazy necks.

Imagine that your head is a bowling ball (the weight of your head and a ball are actually quite similar), and your neck is a stick trying to hold it up. When the head is out of balance by being too far forward, neck and shoulder tightness occurs because the muscles actually have to strain to hold on to the head.

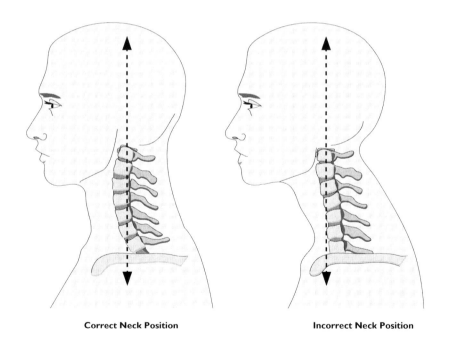

Correct Neck Position   Incorrect Neck Position

Figure 2. Correct vs. incorrect head position.

The extent of the forward head carriage is easily measured by looking at a patient or by taking a lateral (side-view) X-ray of the neck. The farther forward the head, the bigger the problem and the greater the likelihood of developing arthritis and pain in the neck. Stretches, exercises, ergonomic repositioning, and chiropractic adjustment can all be helpful in correcting this postural problem.

The Importance of Flexibility

Flexibility is absolutely vital to our health, but even people who exercise regularly get into a rut. In our offices, we often see the long-distance runner who can't touch his toes. Imagine being fit enough to run 10 or more miles at a time and yet being so tight you can't touch your toes! Even very fit people frequently can't turn their heads in the full range of motion. This is a frightening thought, because one of the most important physical attributes you need when driving a car is the ability to turn your head and look behind you. (Car manufacturers are now adding rear-facing cameras, reducing the need for drivers to turn their heads while driving. Although this is partially to offset the lack of lower rear visibility in big cars, there is no doubt that our population's declining neck mobility adds to the desirability of these cameras.)

Testing for Flexibility

Are you flexible? You need to be. People who age well are people who are flexible, maintain good muscle tone, and work on balance—all vitally important as we grow older—and flexibility is an ability that is easier to hold on to than to regain once you stiffen up as you get older. (Even people in their 20s who don't work out begin to lose flexibility.)

Here are a few tests to see how flexible you are:

- ❑ Can you touch your toes? If not, can you touch your ankles?
- ❑ Can you clap your hands behind your back?
- ❑ Can you drop your chin to your chest?
- ❑ Can you put your head back and look up without it hurting?

- ❏ When you bend to the side, can you touch the sides of your knees?

- ❏ When standing and with your feet pointing ahead of you, extend your arms and twist to the left. Then twist to the right. You ought to be getting to approximately the same point on both sides.

- ❏ Try bending your head to the left; then to the right. Ideally, you want to be able to get your ear almost to your shoulder on each side without moving your shoulder.

Five Tips for Achieving Optimal Flexibility

1. Adopt a safe and effective stretching program. Consistency is key.
Building or maintaining flexibility requires regular stretching. You can't expect to be flexible if you only stretch once in a while. A regular stretching program is essential for achieving and maintaining optimal flexibility, but there's a side benefit: It also provides a moment to de-stress, collect your thoughts, and really pay attention to your body each day.

2. "No pain, no gain" does not apply to stretching.
Pain when stretching means that muscle fibers are strained. These fibers can create scar tissue as the area heals, which increases the risk of problems and stiffness in the future. This is the opposite effect you want to achieve by stretching!

3. Your stretching routine doesn't have to take a long time.
Between 10 and 15 minutes is plenty of time to thoroughly stretch your entire body. Do not rush through stretches. Taking time with each position is effective and reduces the risk of injury.

4. Never end a workout without a stretch.
Many people have the misconception that it is more important to stretch before exercising than it is to stretch after. Actually, stretching too much before working out can increase the risk of straining or tearing your muscles. It is much better to do a light cardio warm-up first and save the more aggressive stretching for afterward. If you do this consistently, you will also reduce any feelings of soreness.

5. Practice balanced stretching.

Stretch each area of the body equally. Stretching one area of the body more than the other can actually do more harm than good by creating an imbalance in your flexibility. A properly constructed stretching program will make sure that each part of the body is stretched correctly. This book offers some excellent suggestions, but there are also very good books on the market that specifically address stretching.

An Ounce of Prevention Is Worth a Pound of Cure

The dentists got it right. The American Dental Association is unified in its approach to oral health for patients of all ages, and there is a standard of care that the public is aware of: Each individual is responsible for daily cleaning, and for optimum health, patients are expected to visit a dentist a couple of times each year for professional cleanings and to get regular dental X-rays to check for cavities.

Dentists don't just sit back and wait until your teeth rot away before they do anything. They continually monitor, preventively treat, and think of new ways to educate you about taking care of your teeth.

What would happen if we took the same approach to our spines and backs?

If we standardized a preventive structural approach to our spines and backs, people would be taking care of one of the most important parts of their bodies—the spine, which holds us erect and protects the spinal cord, through which all our nerves connect, from the head to the organs and limbs. Let's suppose you visited a chiropractor on a regular basis and got some back-strengthening exercises from a physical therapist, which you then performed regularly at home (just like flossing and brushing your teeth). You would be in better health and less likely to suffer back pain!

Scoliosis

Scoliosis is a description of a condition, not a disease in itself. The causes are poorly understood and of unknown origin. If viewed from the back, a normal spine should follow a straight line from your neck all the way down to your buttocks. In scoliosis, the spine grows with a curvature. School nurses and pediatricians check for this condition during the years when children are going through major growth spurts. Though the severity of the curvature is more common in girls, scoliosis can also affect boys. Curvatures are measured by degrees, and the larger the degree of curvature, the greater the consequences. If the curvature of the back is between 0 and 15 degrees, most doctors recommend no treatment whatsoever other than monitoring the curve. In my opinion, this is the equivalent of staring at it while hoping that it won't get any worse. If the curvature of the back is between 15 and 35 degrees, doctors often recommend bracing, in which the patient wears what looks like a body cast to help stop the curvature from worsening. If bracing doesn't work, most physicians recommend surgery, in which metal rods are surgically inserted on both sides of the spine to stabilize it. If you've ever tied a tomato plant to a stake, then you understand the concept of what must be accomplished surgically.

In my experience, doctors believe that a curvature cannot really be changed without surgery. I disagree. There are numerous techniques that can be beneficial to help get a patient's spine in better balance. That is not to say that surgical intervention is always wrong in every case, but the rush to surgery should be eliminated.

I do not pretend to have the cure for scoliosis; however, the following story from a concerned parent offers the possibility that a better approach might be available.

My son George has been getting his spine checked for scoliosis about twice a year since he was very young (once by our pediatrician and once in school). No problems were ever detected. But at age 15, during a regular checkup, George's pediatrician detected what he thought was a "slight" curve. A follow-up X-ray of [George's] back revealed that what we thought was about a 7-degree curve was actually a 27-degree curve!

We quickly took George to an orthopedic surgeon to find out what to do next. I was surprised to find that the doctor did not have many answers for us and recommended that no action be taken in terms of treatment. He said that we could put [George] in a brace, but it would be very uncomfortable and severely limit [his] activity. [The doctor] also told us that even the brace would not do anything to lessen the curve but only prevent [the curve] from worsening.

The thought of just waiting to see if my son's condition worsened was frustrating and frightening. I asked if there was anything that he could change by doing exercises, carrying a different type of bag, or even eating differently. The doctor said no to all of these things.

Out of concern and frustration I decided to seek an alternative opinion and was referred to Midtown Chiropractic [because of] their willingness to explore all the options. Dr. Sinett immediately explained that the right side of George's body was much stronger than the left. He gave [George] exercises to strengthen his transverse abdominal muscles and improve his pos-

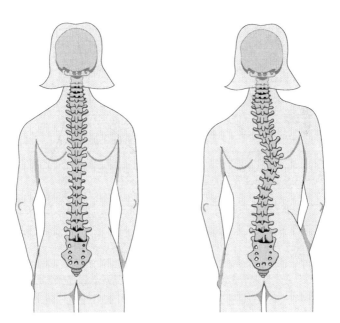

Figure 3. A normal spine compared to a scoliotic spine.

ture. He also explained ways that George's body could become more balanced by improving his nutrition. After two treatments with [the doctor], George was retested with another X-ray, ordered by the same orthopedist, which revealed that his curve was only 17 degrees (10 degrees less than the original!).

While I wouldn't begin to claim that we cured George—or have a cure for scoliosis—the improvement in the measurement was dramatic; and, more important, we provided George with some relief from the pain he was experiencing because of his condition.

CHAPTER 5

A Prescription for Structural Issues

"I don't know what happened. The pain came out of nowhere."

This is one of the most frequent comments we hear from new patients. But back pain doesn't come out of nowhere. There's always a cause. However, I will say this: When it comes to back issues, there is always the proverbial "straw that broke the camel's back." Many minor indignities to your back add up to the point that one significant—or not so significant—thing happens that throws out your back.

Where Does Structural Back Pain Come From?

This question has led to millions of dollars in studies, but in our chiropractic practice, we already have the answer: Barring any sign of trauma or injury, it's the little things that cumulatively contribute to overwhelming back pain. It can be as simple as bad postural habits that accrue to the point that they cause structural back pain.

In Chapter 4, you learned the basics about your back and spine and the possible root of pain caused by structural problems. This chapter shows you how activities in daily life may be creating or contributing to your back pain.

"Prevent the bad-habit buildup" has become one of my mantras. If you recognize yourself in some of the bad habits we discuss in this chapter, then this is your wake-up call to fight off back pain before it gets worse. Our goal here is to prevent the buildup of bad habits that will compound themselves and result in pain. You will see that some relatively simple fixes can have a profound effect.

But before we talk about specific lifestyle issues and bad habits, we first need to talk about two very important issues that affect most of us every single day: the importance of good posture, and backbreaking work.

Good Posture Equals Good Health

The person who exhibits good posture is much less likely than others to suffer back or neck pain. He or she understands the proper way of standing and sitting that promotes a strong back, and this person likely has good spinal flexibility. This flexibility, gained through proper exercise and sometimes aided by chiropractic adjustments, is another key to overall good health because it gives all parts of the body the opportunity to function properly.

But what *is* good posture? Most people really don't know. Is it ramrod-straight posture, like a tin soldier? Are the shoulders and collar bone supposed to be as stretched out as a ballerina's? What about a bodybuilder? Is he the ideal?

The answer is a little of all of these.

When a person is viewed from the side in a standing posture, he should have complete vertical alignment of the ear, shoulder, hip, knee, and ankle. But there is a difference between the relaxed, easy look of someone with good posture, and the forced erectness of a soldier in formation.

The spine is made up of three curves (as shown in Figure 4). These curves develop as we grow, and help us support our spine and provide adequate function and flexibility. When people slip into bad habits from laziness or injury, their slumped posture puts stress on the spine because the spine has trouble supporting the body when it is out of alignment. This imbalance results in dysfunction and can cause varying levels of pain or discomfort. On a so-called minor level, the discomfort is a medium-level headache or back or neck pain, which can mean days off from work or just a general achy feeling. If this misalignment goes on for a prolonged period of time, the body sends in reinforcements by growing

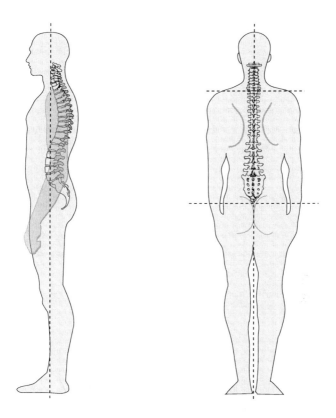

Figure 4. Correct standing posture.

more bone to help with the additional stress. Spinal stenosis or osteoarthritis (a progressive breakdown of cartilage, the tissue that protects and cushions the joints) can result. Eventually, this can lead to bone rubbing on bone, an exceedingly painful condition that can limit a person's overall quality of life.

But bad posture is only one of many ways we do structural damage to our bodies.

A New Definition of Backbreaking Work

Work that used to be described as backbreaking really isn't. Would you believe that farmers in underdeveloped areas where much of the work is done without the benefit of machines have less incidence of back pain than people in developed countries? The real backbreaking jobs are the ones that keep us seated, doing small movements over and over. While a farmer can certainly overdo lifting or pulling, thus creating a sprain or strain injury, farming allows a person to move his or her body in all different directions.

As it happens, one of the main causes of chronic musculoskeletal pain is our sedentary lifestyle. Sitting exerts 30 percent more pressure on your spine than standing, so work that looks light and easy, such as sitting at a desk all day, is actually backbreaking. Most of us further lighten our workload when we use modern conveniences such as washing machines and vacuums and when we rely on cars for getting us around. All these advances have led to humans living very sedentary lifestyles. That's not good for our backs! The repetitive small movements that are part of our new lifestyles are not allowing our body "freeness" in range of motion. Technology has made everything too easy, and our bodies are paying the price.

I call this condition *disuse syndrome*. If you don't give your muscles something to do, they get weaker and smaller. If you sit around, your joints lose lubrication and age faster. If you don't use it or move it, you lose it. And if you don't keep a

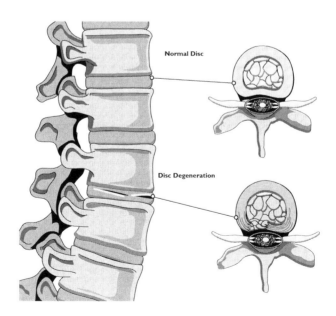

Figure 5. Degeneration of the spine.

healthy, aligned spine, you lose energy and balance, and over time, your joints degenerate.

Numerous studies have shown the benefit of exercise when it comes to back pain: The percentage of people who suffer from back pain is the same as that of people who don't exercise. Norwegian researchers prodded 500 people to exercise daily. They didn't specify the type of exercise or the amount of time the study subjects should devote to it—the instructions were simply to "get moving." The results of the study were quite amazing. The risk of having back pain dropped by 50 percent for those participants who began exercising daily.

Don't be sedentary. Find an enjoyable way to start moving—it should be something you enjoy and something you can commit to doing over time. The commitment to take a daily walk is a good example. I'd rather have patients take on a type of exercise they enjoy and will continue for a lifetime than to choose a more active form that they won't continue. Both running and tennis are great for some people; but for others, this sort of exercise may be too energetic, too time-consuming, or too hard on the joints. Choose something that can become part of your life.

In addition to some regular form of exercise, add extra movements to your daily lifestyle. If you're an office worker, get up every hour; move around and stretch out a bit. Don't let your job or your bad habits become backbreaking.

Improving Your Work Environment

We spend most of our working hours sitting, so learn how to take care of your spine when doing so. As noted earlier in this chapter, sitting exerts 30 percent more pressure on your spine than does standing; unfortunately, most of us spend more time sitting than in any other position. It's the main reason back pain is the number one cause of work-related disability. Between commuting (whether you are the driver or passenger) and the number of hours most of us spend at our desks each day working or engaged in leisure-time activities (lounging in front of the television or hunching over the computer are prime among them), we are in our chairs a lot.

By examining MRI studies and evaluating compressive loads (how much

Ergonomics: Helpful, but Not the Whole Answer

Ergonomics is the study of the mechanics of the workplace and analyzes how best to set up workstations to fit the proper job function. Work conditions are definitely better now that both furniture designers and the workers themselves understand the importance of ergonomic correctness, and these alterations in the workplace have prevented many types of repetitive strain injuries, saving employees millions of dollars in reduced sick time. This is all well and good, but it is no cure-all.

Our problem with ergonomics is that it places the emphasis on engineering furniture when we ought to be emphasizing the human body and keeping it in balance. The core imbalance is behind most of the problems that make the ergonomic industry so profitable. Therefore, we're for eliminating the cause altogether by eliminating the core imbalance so that your working life will be more comfortable and your risk of injury will be diminished. A body in balance is a healthy body.

weight is put where in our bodies), researchers in Scotland found that sitting up straight (at a 90-degree angle) can put much strain on the body. The pressure of an upright seated position compresses the discs and can cause them to become misaligned, often resulting in considerable back pain.

These researchers noted that by sitting at a 135-degree angle, it was possible to alleviate much of the compressive load. (This angle is formed when your feet are on the floor but your torso is angled back a bit.) By leaning back, your back muscles are permitted to relax, and the space in your chest opens a bit. Although this may not be practical when working at a computer (and more about that in a moment), most people have idle moments—phone time, thinking time, coworker-stops-by-your-desk time—when they can shift positions (stand or lean back in their chair) to give their back muscles a rest. The study also identified that the worst posture to be in for prolonged periods is a seated position, slouching forward, which dramatically increases the compression on chest and spine.

If you don't have a desk chair that lets you tilt back safely now and then,

Simple Stretches, Big Relief

1. If you've been sitting for an hour, stand up and walk around, then put your hands on your buttocks (palm on the buttocks, fingers pointing down) and stretch back (your arms should be akimbo and will stretch back like chicken wings).

2. Clasp your hands together behind you and pull down, keeping hands together, then stretch them back behind you. You can enhance this stretch by bending forward at the hips, keeping your arms stretched out behind you, hands clasped. Let the weight of your arms pull your arms (stretched straight) toward the floor. This simple maneuver releases a great deal of tension.

3. Sitting upright, place your right hand over your head, just above your left ear. Apply pressure gently to the right for about 10 seconds, stretching the left side of your neck. Repeat the same gentle pull with your left hand by your right ear. Do this twice on each side and repeat periodically throughout the day.

you should think about buying one. And when you drive, consider positioning the seat so that your back tilts back slightly—it can tilt back even more when you're the passenger. How about when you're relaxing at home? Recliners allow you to tilt your back in a way that takes pressure off the spine; at the same time, they provide support for the legs and head—a perfect postural solution for sitting.

Correct Posture While at Work

Here's what you need to know about sitting where most of us spend hours each day—at our desks or in front of a computer screen.

A proper chair is one that maintains all your spinal curves when sitting. This means that your lower back should be supported, and your head should be able to be basically straight when looking toward the computer monitor. Purchase a desk chair (or at the office, ask for this type of chair) that provides lower

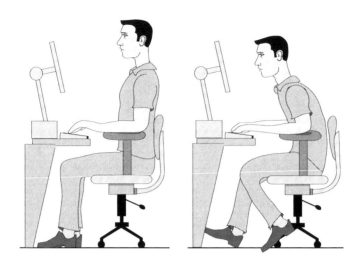

Figure 6. Correct vs. incorrect office chair position.

back (lumbar) support. If your workplace is unlikely to buy you a new chair, purchase a pillow that supports your lower back and place it behind you on the chair.

The chair itself should be on wheels so that you can pull yourself into a comfortable work position with feet resting lightly on the floor or, for a shorter person, on a stool underneath the desk.

If you have to bend forward to use the keyboard, or if your neck must crane forward to see the monitor, you will experience back and neck strain. Monitors today are highly adjustable, so if yours seems too high or too low, shift the position so that it feels right to you. If it's an old monitor and is sitting lower than is comfortable, grab something (an old phone book is ideal) to raise it up.

Don't Just Sit There

For every muscle that you have in your body, there is another muscle that works in opposition. It's sort of a yin and yang throughout the body, allowing you to bend both forward and backward, for example. When you get stuck in one position for too long, it throws off the important muscular yin and yang of contract and relax. To keep your muscles in balance, do the following:

- Shift your weight every few minutes. Arch your back, lean back, lean forward, shift from side to side.

- When you get a phone call, stand up for at least part of the time you are talking; shift your weight from one foot to the other until you hang up or have to sit down again.

- About every 30 minutes, get up and walk around for a couple of minutes—get supplies, change the printer paper, or get up for a drink of water.

Carpal Tunnel and Improved Posture

In addition to back pain, my patients frequently complain of carpal tunnel syndrome, a painful progressive condition caused by compression of a key nerve in the wrist. This pain in the wrist area can actually be caused by nerve compression in the neck, which blocks the flow of nutrients to the nerves in the wrist. Good posture—coupled with appropriate exercise of the arms, shoulders, and wrists—can help stop carpal tunnel syndrome from developing in the first place.

The current approach to treatment for carpal tunnel syndrome is bracing the wrists, taking anti-inflammatory medications, and undergoing physical therapy. If those methods are ineffective, then doctors usually recommend surgery. However, as a professional who sees a lot of the "nothing is helping" cases, I recommend that you try out all noninvasive possibilities—including chiropractic—before signing up for surgery. A chiropractic adjustment, physical therapy, or improved posture may help increase blood flow to the arm and wrist and thus reduce pain. Patients who concentrate on improving their posture have a general decrease in stress-related symptoms, including carpal tunnel syndrome.

Sitting Pretty

Because sitting is hard on the body—and because we often don't have a choice as to what type of seating is offered to us throughout our day—here are some other solutions to maintaining a healthy back in seats that are bad for us.

- **BAR STOOLS** (in kitchens as well as at bars). Good posture and bar stools do *not* go hand in hand. Because most people curl over and lean on the bar or counter, they reinforce the "compression factor" (see Chapter 6). Instead, sit up on the stool, with your pelvis tipped forward slightly. The waist is not a hinge, so don't bend there. If your feet are suspended, rest them on a rail under the stool. Women tend to put additional strain on the hips while fighting to keep their legs together when seated on these high stools.

- **RESTAURANT BOOTHS**. These are manageable if they are narrow enough to let you lean back or if they are firm enough that you can perch forward; again, pelvis tilted forward with the shoulders back. Ideally, restaurants with bench seating will provide pillows that you can place behind your back, allowing diners to "custom-fit" their seat.

- **MOLDED SEATS** (the type on buses and in some restaurants). These are designed to crunch the pelvis toward the torso, which is definitely

Reading and Back/Neck Pain

Reading can be hard on the neck! If you put the book in your lap, your neck is placed at a tough angle for a prolonged period of time. Instead, find a way to elevate your reading material. In bed or on a couch, put a pillow in your lap so your arms and the book are elevated. At the office, place the book on the desk so that it's easy to see looking straight on instead of looking down. Specialty catalogs offer book supports that permit you to prop a book on a table for hands-free reading. This positioning is usually preferable for the neck.

not good for you. If you're forced to sit on one of these, perch forward and sit up straight.

- **THE COUCH.** Couches can be great places to curl up, but it is healthier for your spine if you take time to prop the pillows behind you in such a way that you can create support for your back. Remember a slight backward tilt is ideal

Correcting Other Bad Habits and Improving Lifestyle Issues

Over time we all slip into bad habits that can contribute to back pain. But there are some lifestyle choices that we can make to improve not only our back health but our overall well-being.

Improve Your Sleeping Environment

Choose a Proper Mattress

Mattresses are so big and so heavy that once you have one, you really don't want to think about tossing it out and getting a new one, the way you might a new set of towels. Manufacturers assert that mattresses should be replaced on a regular basis; this claim is backed up by household hints guru Heloise, who notes that mattresses actually do wear out, most lasting only 8 to 10 years. The lifetime of a mattress is affected by the weight of the occupants and their lifestyle habits: Do two Labrador retrievers share the bed with you? Do you sit on the mattress a lot during the day? Do the kids jump on it (without your approval, I hope)?

Although no one likes having to make major expenditures, don't begrudge buying a new mattress every 10 years or so. Mattress manufacturing keeps getting better and better. In addition, our understanding of what makes a good mattress has changed over the years. If you bought a mattress as recently as 10 years ago, chances are the salesperson told you that a firm mattress was best for your back. Today, we know that rock-hard mattresses are actually not at all good for the back, and they aren't conducive to a good night's sleep, either.

A study published in the highly respected British medical journal the *Lancet* followed 313 adults who had chronic lower back pain. The subjects were divided into two groups. Half slept on a firm mattress, and the other half slept on a medium-firm mattress for 90 days. Researchers were surprised to learn that those who slept on the medium-firm mattresses had less pain than the other group. They surmised that the medium-firm mattresses may have been better because they gave support but also conformed to the body, which proved to be less stressful for the spine.

To determine whether you should be in the market for a new mattress, you need to listen to your body. If you are waking up tight and stiff every morning, consider whether your mattress is the culprit.

As a matter of fact, a recent study conducted by Oklahoma State University researchers and reported in the *Journal of Chiropractic Medicine* revealed that subjects who suffered from persistent back pain found immediate and significant relief by switching to a new mattress and that the improvements persisted past the initial switch. The study also found that subjects who slept on mattresses that were at least 5 years old were significantly more likely to suffer from back pain and stiffness. It is interesting that subjects who suffered the greatest back pain reported a significant improvement in back discomfort after switching mattresses.

Do you need a new mattress? Consider the following ABCs:

- **A (AGE).** Has your mattress had more than 8 years of nightly use?

- **B (BEAUTY).** Does your mattress have stains, soil, or tears? Does it sag?

- **C (COMFORT).** When you lie down and concentrate on the comfort of your mattress, does it feel good or is it beginning to hollow out and sag in places?

In addition, try this support test: Lie flat on your back on your current mattress or the mattress you are considering buying. Place your hand under the small of your back. How much space is there? (You should be able to move your hand around.)

If you resolve to buy a new mattress, go to a store, listen to the salesperson, and test out a few models. (If you have a sleeping partner, shop together so that you can both test it.) Remove your shoes and lie down on several different mattress models, testing out various positions, especially the position you usually sleep in. Pay special attention to the support of your lower back and your postural alignment (as if you were standing), and make sure you feel plenty of comfort at the shoulders and hips. A few extra minutes spent paying attention to the feel of different mattresses can be time well spent.

Before making a purchase, check out the store's return policy. A mattress is a big investment. Just because you lie on one in the store and it seems comfortable, there is no guarantee that it will be the one that works for you at night. The store that has a good return policy and will allow you to take a mattress for a test drive is the right place to buy.

During the 30-day trial period, listen to your body. Do you wake up feeling relaxed and refreshed? Do you feel as if you had a good night's sleep? Just like Goldilocks, you need to find the mattress that is just right. If you don't feel great when you wake up, then it's not the right mattress for you. Send it back.

And once you are satisfied, remember that mattresses do require some tending. Purchase a cotton mattress cover for it. In addition, mattress professionals say it's important to rotate and reverse the mattress about every 6 months to even out the wear.

Pillow Talk

Since the late 1990s, the importance of a proper pillow has gained media attention, but in our office, we've known it for years. At least now we're getting some help from marketers who are reminding people that the proper pillow can prevent neck and back pain and an improper one can actually be the source of discomfort.

When you sleep, your head should lie slightly lower than your neck so that both your head and neck musculature are at rest. When you sleep on a standard pillow, your head receives most of the support while the muscles of your neck must work to hold the head in position during sleep. Based on this fact, manufacturers created what they called a "chiropractic pillow," which had a bump at neck level and a scooped-out area for the head. If you went to sleep and never moved, then both your head and lower neck would be supported. But, given how active we all are during our sleep—shifting, turning, moving about—you have to wonder, what *were* they thinking? Fortunately, pillows have improved over the years.

Owing to the development of new materials, memory pillows and other designs intended to prevent back and neck pain are currently on the market. My personal choice, however, is a water pillow. Yes, a water pillow. Water is dynamic, so no matter how you move, the supportive aspects of the pillow adjust right with you. As a result, your head will always be lower than your neck. The result is perfect posture while you are sleeping. This is the type of pillow my family and I sleep on, and it is the pillow that I recommend for my patients.

When I take a patient's history, I ask about pillow types and sleeping habits. Often people tell me they sleep with multiple pillows. Your neck needs to be at the proper angle at which it can be at rest; when you use more than one pillow, the angle of your neck creates stress, which prevents the area from relaxing.

One of the most common pillow-related bad habits is reading or watching television in bed. Comfy as it is when you start out, this "crunched" posture can unfortunately lead to trouble later on (see Chapter 6 for more on core imbalance). Too much forward bending in your neck can easily be the cause of your back pain.

Promote Spinal Health While You Sleep

The best gift you can give your body is a good night's sleep, and the combination of the correct mattress and the correct pillow can make a big difference to your health.

Your sleeping posture should maintain all of the curves of the spine—the neck, the mid-back, and the lower back. And you should support those curves on a good pillow and a medium-firm mattress.

How to Sleep

Our patients often ask, "What is a proper sleeping position?" They wonder if they should sleep on their back, side, or stomach.

If you are able to fall asleep, that generally means you are comfortable. If we prescribed a particular sleep position, your sleep would likely be disrupted. The last thing you want to worry about when dozing off is trying to stay in a specific position. However, if you are suffering from back pain, here are the ideal sleep positions:

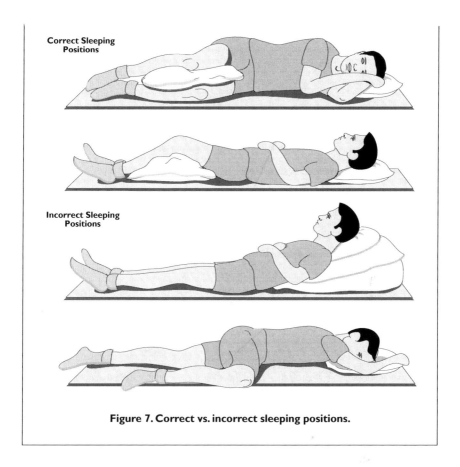

Figure 7. Correct vs. incorrect sleeping positions.

The Shoulder "Phone Clamp"

It used to be that my typical patient who had pain from using the phone was an office worker—usually an administrative assistant, a stockbroker, or a reporter. These people sat at their desks most of the day cradling the phone between their shoulder and ear—a terrible thing to do to your neck.

Today I have many more phone-pain patients, and their pain is worse than that of my patients from earlier in my career. Why? Because more people than ever are talking on the phone—on trains, in cars, and on the street, as well as in homes and offices—and the phones are getting smaller and smaller. The smaller the phone, the greater the neck crunch necessary to clench the phone between shoulder and ear. This simple move, when done repetitively, can easily rob you of flexibility in your neck, resulting in pain. When people do the clamp maneuver to free their hands while they talk, they intensify the tension in the neck and shoulder area.

The solution is quite simple. Make sure you are not holding the phone between your neck and shoulder. Wear a headset whenever possible. The very simple act of holding the phone with your arm tightens a good number of muscles, and while it is not as debilitating as the shoulder clamp, prolonged phone use can still cause long-term pain. (If you use a phone while driving, invest in a hands-free system to save your back—and perhaps your life!)

Credit-Carditis: More Than Bad Debt

Just as a crooked foundation is disastrous for a building, so, too, is an uneven foundation damaging for the spine. The pelvis, the lowermost part of the spine, is like the foundation of a house, and the head, neck, and shoulders are the upper floors. If your pelvis is not aligned properly, it can easily cause damage to your hips, lower back, and even your neck.

Men who carry their wallets in their back pocket sit on an uneven surface all day, throwing off the balance of their lower spine. This problem was first identified as "credit-carditis" in a report that appeared in the *New England Journal of Medicine* in 1966.

The slight change in the position of the pelvic bones causes a stretching of tissues on one side of the body and a shortening and contracting on the other. Because the pelvis's biomechanics must adapt to the change in balance, the rest of the body must compensate as well. Although the onset is gradual, the continued pressure by an object that presses on the piriformis muscle in the buttocks (which is connected to the sciatic nerve) can result in pain that radiates throughout the back and hip area. It doesn't take long for such subtle changes to affect the body.

Your gait and your standing posture may be altered by the changes that have occurred from sitting on your wallet. (Golfers who stuff balls into their back pockets suffer the same problem, caused by the balls pressing against their buttocks muscle for prolonged periods.) Your body has the amazing capacity to reverse these negative changes when you stand up. However, if you sit on your wallet for 8 to 10 hours a day and you have been doing so for many years, your body may begin to lose the ability to self-correct.

There's a relatively simple solution: Put your money in a money clip in a front pocket. If you wear a suit, your credit cards could go in a slim wallet in an inner front-jacket pocket. If you're not a suit-and-tie guy and need to carry a wallet in your back pocket, then open it up and remove all the artifacts you've been carrying around. When I have people do this in the office, they often discover out-of-date health insurance cards, reward and membership cards that they haven't used in years, not to mention a variety of credit cards that are used only very occasionally. Cut down on what you carry, and treat yourself to a lightweight, thin wallet if you must carry one; preferably, however, you should find another way to carry your money and cards.

Loosen Up (Your Clothing)

Researchers have found that there is a direct link between tight clothing and numerous health issues. This issue dates back to Renaissance times when women wore corsets. Women used to have fainting spells after being laced into these contraptions. Today, our clothing is not quite that constricting, but super-tight garments do restrict one's breathing, which is not healthy. Wearing clothing that is too tight can also cause stomach pain, groin pain, and shortness of breath, and can even lower sperm counts.

It is surprising to note that it's not just women in body-hugging jeans who are suffering. In my offices, I often find that men who have put on a little weight are squeezing themselves into old pants—and belts—that are just too tight. Clothing that is worn too tight can even mimic a hernia. Billy Crystal's *Saturday Night Live* character was mistaken when he said it was more important to look good than to feel good.

Swallow your pride and loosen your belt. If you follow the diet suggestions given in Part III, you'll likely find that you can go back to the tighter notch on your belt in a couple of months.

Lighten Your Load

In the last couple of years, fashionable handbags have become mini-suitcases, and women's shoulders and backs are suffering. Some of the bags themselves are heavy, but the large size of the bag permits women to load up on what they carry, and the weight adds up! This has become an important enough issue that in 2006 the *New York Times* ran an article about it, and the American Chiropractic Association has drawn up guidelines for what to do about women's handbags.

The most noticeable side effect of a too-heavy purse is that a woman's shoulders become uneven. In order to tote the weighty purse on her arm or carry it as a shoulder bag, the woman actually elevates the working shoulder, which throws both her spine and overall sense of balance out of whack. (It's even worse if she's also using a cell phone without a headset.)

This kind of damage can be comparable to a painful sports injury, and if not remedied, it can create a long-term back problem. Women frequently visit chiropractors, and some report going to doctors for cortisone shots because of the pain of a too-big purse. That's crazy.

Most women aren't going to give up carrying handbags, so here are some recommendations:

- The American Chiropractic Association recommends that a handbag weigh no more than 10 percent of its owner's body weight. I would put forward that even a bag that weighs "only" 10 percent of your body weight can still be an awfully heavy bag to carry every day.

- When you select a bag, be certain the bag itself is a lightweight one. At this writing, fashionable purses are decorated with heavy chains and metal locks, and the extra weight adds up.

- Clean your handbag out once a week, and empty your coins regularly. Both these practices will be a big help in keeping the bag at a manageable weight.

- Try switching hands or shoulders when carrying a handbag. This will provide you with a more balanced "work out."

- Consider carrying both a handbag and a briefcase. A lightweight shoulder purse that holds just a few items can be balanced by a briefcase carried on the other side of the body; this distributes the weight more evenly and still allows you to carry all your necessities.

Men and Children, Too!

Men and children should also pay attention to what they carry. Men can be well served by paring down the contents of their briefcases and gym bags. Children need help with selecting a lightweight backpack and then packing judiciously. (Parents may need to supervise the regular cleaning out of a younger child's backpack to be sure it gets done.) Some school systems have become aware of the harm children sustain from carrying too much in their backpacks, and some districts provide each student with two copies of their textbooks—one to keep at school and one to have at home. This can greatly ease the load on the backs of our growing children. Some parents have successfully gotten their children to use backpacks on wheels; if your child is willing to use one, it's a good option.

The Back Belt—Helpful or Not?

People who do a lot of lifting for a living frequently wear back belts or braces, and this is also a habit that some weekend warriors have adopted because they think it will help them do certain kinds of exercises—particularly heavy lifting—that they wouldn't normally be able to do.

Back belts are actually more of a hindrance than a benefit because they affect proprioception, which is a five-dollar word for something that restricts your brain's ability to get messages from other parts of your body. Wearing a belt can impede the messages that your back is trying to tell your brain, such as "Take a break," "Ease off," or "Don't lift this! It's too heavy!"

A back belt is like an ice pack. If you get hurt, the back belt can give your back a break and protect it for a little while. But once you're past a crisis period, it's important to get back to relying on your own musculature.

Bad Shoes Create Bad Backs

Your back would like you to walk in low-heeled shoes (they don't have to be totally flat) that permit your weight to be balanced across the ball and the heel of your foot. Your feet—and your back—are also happiest if your foot fits snugly in the shoe and stays there. (Business in chiropractic offices skyrockets in the summer months when both men and women start wearing sandals and flip-flops.)

To avoid back pain caused by foot imbalances, you may want to reconsider spending the weekend wearing flip-flops or trekking to work in backless high heels. These styles lead to foot instability. A backless shoe allows your foot to slide from side to side, distributing your body's weight in an uneven manner. High heels cause your foot to strike the ground in a more toe-forward motion, which can jar your knees, hips, and lower back. When you combine this with the instability of an open-back shoe, the joint and back pain at the end of the day can be twofold!

I'm definitely not saying that you should never wear stylish shoes. But when you are doing a lot of walking and standing, consider sandals with backs and buckling straps or laces, and lower-heeled shoes with some arch support. Your feet are happiest—and both back and feet are healthiest—when you are in a shoe that provides even support and firmly holds your foot in place when you walk. Lace-up shoes are ideal, but there are more fashionable styles that accomplish this same purpose. I realize that some of these shoes do not provide the most elegant look, so here are two tips for choosing a shoe when you have to think about a little more than function:

- A woman's dress shoe should have a supportive back and a snug (not tight) fit that holds the foot in place.

- The best casual sandals are those made especially for outdoor activity. The more support the better. (Several companies make sandals that offer enough support that you can run in them—and they still look fashionable).

Exercise Habits

Though the next chapter is fully devoted to exercising to build a strong core, the following are some of the key elements to consider when exercising.

Warming Up Before Exercise Is Important

The ideal workout is broken into three equal parts: warm-up, training, and cool-down. (A 30-minute workout becomes 10-10-10.) This simple method removes the shock factor to your muscular system and back. By warming up properly, your muscles will be more flexible, and greater flexibility will prevent injuries.

Using the Treadmill

Treadmills are a fine way to exercise because they guarantee that you can get moving, rain or shine, dawn or night. But remember: The goal of the treadmill experience is simply to keep moving at a normal gait—not too fast, not too slow—arms swinging. Unfortunately, people misuse this machine in ways that can cause injury.

The most common mistake that people make when using a treadmill is having the platform elevated. The rationale for this is that by raising the platform and creating an uphill stride, the exercise is more intense and the heart rate is elevated. However, when running on an incline, the balance of the body is completely changed. There is a specific biomechanical process that occurs during the normal human gait. Recall that the heel strikes the floor first, then the full foot contacts the floor, followed by a lift off from the forefoot and toes that propels the body forward. This same process offers the proper biomechanics of running. But by raising the platform, the normal biomechanics are altered, forcing some areas of the feet to take on more pressure than they are designed to absorb and leaving other areas of the feet underused. In essence, the gait becomes less efficient, and injuries are more likely to occur. Of course, we all walk up and down inclines and declines every day. However, running on a treadmill with a steep incline creates unrelenting imbalance—and the pain and injuries that follow.

The second most common misuse of the treadmill is walking or running at a faster pace than you can properly handle. Find a comfortable speed at which you can maintain a normal stride (not too short and not too long).

If you find that you have to hold on to the side rails, then you are not walking or running at the best pace. When you walk or run, you are not just using your feet and legs but the entire body. When you take a step forward with the right leg, the left arm swings forward and the body rotates to maintain momentum. This is part of the normal gait pattern, which allows opposing muscles to contract and relax, enabling us to move forward with efficiency and ease. Short-circuiting the walking or running stride by holding on to a rail not only will change the gait pattern but can also lead to injury.

Walking

While proper walking form is generally instinctive, many people have—by training, injury, or other circumstances—fallen into bad habits. It's simple to keep in mind: right leg forward, left arm forward; left leg forward, right arm forward. Your arms swing freely, bent but relaxed at the elbows. This natural motion allows for proper torsion in your mid-back. At the same time, you want to keep your knees relaxed to absorb the impact of each step, head up to avoid neck strain, and shoulders squared with a slight forward roll. The idea is to keep good form but stay relaxed to avoid strain.

This form should stay the same while running or exercising. And if you choose to run or walk on a machine, choose exercise equipment that allows this form. Learn to walk properly before you begin running regularly.

Running

Because running can potentially have some real consequences to your back health, here are some good pointers to remember.

Humans are essentially quadrupeds, meaning that we use all four limbs when we walk or run. And there is a natural synchronous distribution of muscles when we walk or run. When we take a step forward with the right leg, the left arm moves forward while the right arm swings back. This harmonious firing of muscles propels the body forward efficiently.

For every muscle contraction, there is an equal muscle relaxation. For example, as one leg moves forward, the muscle group (called the quadriceps) contracts as the back leg muscle (called the hamstring) relaxes. If they both fired at the same time, you wouldn't be able to move forward.

If the timing of the contracting and relaxing isn't firing right due to improper gait or core imbalance, the result can be muscle strains, sprains, pulls, and tears—and pain. The solution is to learn good form.

And one final piece of advice: Don't run on the sand.

Many people believe that running on the beach is a good workout because it takes more effort than running on a solid surface. But running on sand can lead to injury. Because of the erosion from the water, the beach tends to slope, so this throws off a runner's normal running gait. And if you are running on softer sand, your feet are not getting a firm surface to strike and then toe off from. The uneven surface throws off your balance and creates myriad symptoms, including foot pain; shin splints; and knee, hip, and back pain. If you want to run by the beach, do it on the boardwalk!

CHAPTER 6

Core Imbalance

At first glance, the administrative assistant and the fitness trainer who both visited our offices appeared to have nothing in common. Tracy, a middle-aged office worker, spent a minimum of 40 hours a week at her desk, bent over a computer or crunched up taking phone messages. Her commute to and from the office put her on a city bus for about 25 minutes each morning and evening. Though she suffered from asthma, she still made time to exercise regularly. When she came to our office, she was looking for help with lower back pain.

Kyle offered a sharp contrast to Tracy. He was a fitness trainer in his early 30s who spent all day at a gym teaching fitness, conducting spin classes, and guiding people through individualized workout regimens. His daily life was far from sedentary. When he came to us, it was for help with back and shoulder pain as well as debilitating migraine headaches.

Two totally different patients with very different symptoms, yet just one diagnosis: core imbalance. Both of these people spent too much time working their abs, albeit in very different ways. While Tracy's job doesn't sound like it entails much abdominal work, the very act of being curled up (at a computer, at a desk, or on a bus) meant that her abdomen was in an almost constant state of crunch, her muscles contracted for much of the day. Kyle was actually performing several types of exercises (sit-ups, crunches, curling over a bike in spinning class, and so on) that caused his abdominal muscles to contract but that wasn't good, either. Whether a patient's abs are pulled tight because of bad posture, long periods of sitting, or physical exercise, the results are the same. Tracy and Kyle developed symptoms that resulted from spending too much time with their abdomens compressed.

After diagnosis, we gave each of them advice on how to overcome core imbalance and recommended particular abdominal exercises that would maintain core strength and help correct the imbalance without contributing to the core imbalance.

We were able to see progress with both patients quite quickly. Tracy's back pain went away, and—much to her amazement, though not ours—her asthma improved. In the process of learning to put some space in her chest, she began to breathe more deeply, and this meant that she was less frequently affected by asthma symptoms. As for Kyle, he later wrote to us, saying: "My headaches and shoulder pain are gone. In the process of working with you, I had to relearn everything I had known about abs. Instead of working only on compression with my clients, I now teach everyone about expansion."

Two Abdominal Core Issues That Affect All of Our Patients

There are two major issues that directly affect the back, and both arise from misuse of the abdominals:

- **FOR EVERY FORWARD MOVEMENT, THERE NEEDS TO BE A COUNTER MOVEMENT.** Think of it as the yin and yang (two opposite but complementary forces) of the muscle system. We spend so much time bending forward, working at the computer, walking with poor posture, and doing exercises like crunches that it's vital to our back health that we find ways to counter the forward crunch of these activities to maintain a balanced core.

- **EVERY TIME YOU CONTRACT A MUSCLE, YOU NEED TO BE SURE TO RELAX IT.** Through stress or bad habit, many people contract certain muscles but never allow them the opportunity to relax. Bodybuilders are frequently incapable of turning their heads fully because their muscles are so tight, it's as if they were in a straitjacket. Think about how tight your neck can feel after an unpleasant business meeting; it's very difficult to let those muscles release. You need to find ways to relax your muscles.

What Is Core Imbalance?

Core imbalance is the term we use to describe a condition of excessive compression, which results in the spine curving forward in a C-like shape. When a person suffers from core imbalance, gravity is essentially winning the battle between forward bending and standing up straight. The elderly often endure this problem, even before it is diagnosed as osteoporosis.

Core imbalance can be caused by many everyday activities, such as sitting at a computer, reading in bed, or driving a car. What's more alarming, it can be self-imposed on our quest for six-pack abs by doing exercises such as crunches or other improper core training. All these things lead to compression and compaction.

Most people in today's workforce are also at risk for core imbalance. From dentists, truck drivers, and maintenance workers to photographers, plumbers, and cosmetologists, people spend much of their time crouched over something. Younger people are just starting to experience the long-term effects of poor posture. In the next 10 to 15 years, we are going to have a generation with unprecedented postural problems as a result of their sedentary lifestyles and the enormous amount of time they spend looking at glowing screens at home and at work.

Our patients also include some highly trained athletes who, unfortunately, have never been introduced to the importance of a balanced core. Cyclists, for example, spend hours hunched over their handlebars. If they don't stretch properly afterward, these athletes will suffer core imbalance later on.

Symptoms of Core Imbalance

Tension headaches; temporomandibular joint (TMJ) problems; stiff neck; elbow, wrist, and arm pain; knee pain; lower back pain; dizziness; difficulty breathing; and poor digestion are just a few of the complaints arising from core imbalance. It can even lead to arthritis and degeneration of the spine.

Compression and Expansion Every Single Day

When your chest is open and uplifted, as it is when you are sitting up straight, your heart, lungs, and other bodily systems have less pressure on them, and you experience an increase in oxygen intake, improved blood and lymph supply, better digestion, better flexibility, and an overall improvement in health.

With regular use of the anti-core-imbalance exercises, you should being to feel an expansion of the chest that is very healthy. Getting rid of your core imbalance may also make you taller. It is not uncommon for patients to gain an inch after undergoing treatment for core imbalance because their spines are straighter and they are simply standing up taller.

Treatments for Core Imbalance

We have a two-tiered approach to correcting core imbalance: The first is a very simple process that involves a back-opening method that can *reverse* the years of forward compression. The second involves a series of core exercises that will help you create a balanced six-pack.

Arch Your Way to Feeling Better

To correct the all-too-common way people hunch forward as they sit, walk, and work, we looked for an easy way to open up the chest and back to reverse the posture that is causing pain. The method we developed involves nothing more complicated than lying on a back support for 2 to 3 minutes to let the spine curve backward slightly, extending and loosening the back muscles, opening the chest, and permitting deeper breathing.

This can be done on an exercise ball (also called a physio ball or Swiss ball), which looks like an oversize beach ball. These are available in most fitness centers and can be purchased at a sporting-goods store. However, the ball lacks stability, which is ironically one of its benefits when doing certain kinds of exercise. But you can make a more stable support simply by rolling up a beach towel to create a cylinder about 12 inches long and 4 to 5 inches in diameter, depending on your current level of flexibility. Place the towel on the floor, then lie down with the towel in line with your spine and allow your head to rest on the floor but with no strain on the neck.

When lying on the support, extend both of your hands above your head, allowing the maximum amount of stretch and chest opening. If this is uncomfortable, place your hands behind your head or across your chest. Your comfort is important. (*Note:* People with heart problems, postural hypotension, or dizziness should consult their physician before doing this exercise.)

Do this back and chest opening exercise for just 30 seconds the first time, gradually increasing the time to about 2 minutes each day. If 30 seconds is too difficult, then place a small pillow under your head to ease the stretch a bit. It is important that you progress through the phases slowly to avoid injury. As you feel more comfortable, you can increase the diameter of the towel. After you have spent the requisite time in the stretch, roll off the towel and lie on your side for 1 or 2 minutes. Then stand up gradually to avoid dizziness.

The Arch

In our practice we are using the prototype of a product called the Arch, which was designed to give you the best results for a back opening and stretching exercise. See the end of the book for more details or go online to www.thetruth aboutbackpainbook.com for details.

The Purpose of the Abdominals

Although many people think about working their abs or flattening their stomach, no one ever really stops to think about the actual purpose of these muscles.

The abdomen runs from the groin, or pelvic region, to the bottom of the ribs. For our bodies to function well, our abdominal muscles need to remain open and stretched, as space within the abdomen is vital to good health. The more expansion we are able to create in the abdomen, the more deeply we can breathe, permitting our lungs to take in more oxygen. In addition, most of our digestive process takes place within the abdomen.

The abdominal muscles include three groups:

- **THE TRANSVERSE ABDOMINUS**. This is a flat, triangular muscle that pulls the abdominal wall inward and acts as an internal girdle to stabilize the spine. It is the key to our core stability.

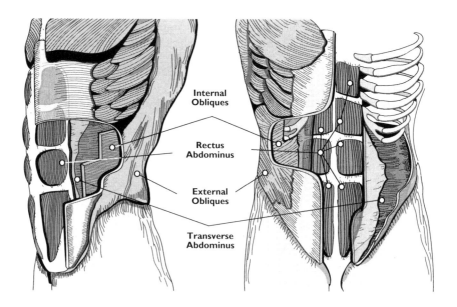

Figure 8. A view of the abdominal muscles.

■ **THE RECTUS ABDOMINUS.** This muscle is responsible for allowing us to bend our trunks forward; it also brings the ribs closer to the pubic bone. This is the muscle that gets overworked from crunching postures and activities. It has no stabilizing effect on the back.

■ **THE INTERNAL AND EXTERNAL OBLIQUES.** These muscles permit us to twist our trunk; the external oblique muscle is the outermost muscle that covers the side of the abdomen. The internal oblique muscle is smaller and thinner than the external and lies just within the external one, providing extra support for side-to-side movements.

Overexercising or underexercising any one of these muscles can cause an imbalance, which can eventually result in pain.

Six Myths About Abdominal Muscles

Myth 1: Strong abs mean a strong back.

"I need to strengthen my abs" is a statement we hear almost every day. But in reality, it's doubtful that your abdominal muscles are weak in relation to the rest of your body. Rather, the problem is more likely that they are not in balance with the rest of your muscles.

Your abs are likely *too strong*, not too weak—even if you don't exercise regularly.

If you spend your day hunched over, the abdominal muscles will be contracted and tight, not stretched and loose. They aren't weak—they are actually too tight.

The heavy emphasis on working your abs comes from a gross misunderstanding of what constitutes good health. The fitness industry makes a fortune selling devices for spot weight reduction (devices or methods that promise to help people get rid of the fat from one part of their bodies, such as the belly or the thighs). And trainers everywhere still recommend sit-ups and crunches as the key to obtaining a flat stomach. But the exercises and devices often featured in infomercials reinforce the false belief that by working out just one part of your body you will receive great benefits.

If you think about it, you *know* this is wrong; you need overall body fitness to be healthy. The truth about all these methodologies lies in the fine-print disclaimer that accompanies most exercise equipment: "This product is effective only when used as part of a complete diet and exercise routine."

The key to a strong back is *balanced* abdominal muscles. Sure, you can work your abs, but no more and no less than you work your other muscles throughout the day. In our work, we've found that proper core balance must come first. If you correct the imbalance, it will correct the weakness and alleviate the symptoms.

Myth 2: A big gut is a sign of weak abs.

A T-shirt I recently saw in an airport sums it up comically: "This isn't a beer belly—just a protective covering for my rock-hard abs!" Big bellies indicate a high percentage of body fat but tell us nothing about abdominal muscle strength or weakness. Sumo wrestlers and large football players—and even some beer drinkers—don't have weak cores. These muscles may be covered with excess fat, but the muscles themselves may be quite strong.

Myth 3: Six-pack abs reflect good abdominal training.

Six-pack abs reflect nice-*looking* muscles, not necessarily properly functioning muscles. It is not uncommon that people with great-looking abs actually suffer pain from imbalance.

Myth 4: Good form while doing abdominal exercises is the best way to protect your neck from injury.

After years of treating patients, I am confident that sit-ups and crunches can be the worst exercises. A common injury sustained during these exercises is "throwing" your neck out. This was first thought to occur when a person didn't support his or her neck, but that couldn't be farther from the truth. Crunches and sit-ups cause the abdominal muscles to be pulled too tight, as if you were wearing a straitjacket. This excessive pulling puts tremendous stress on your neck, and *this* is what "throws" your neck out.

Myth 5: Pilates is a safe, low-impact way to exercise your stomach because it stretches and lengthens the spine, thus preventing injuries.

While a lot of people swear by Pilates, the exercises can cause injuries, and we have a good number of Pilates teachers as patients. The Pilates Hundred exercise—done in almost every class—places an overemphasis on developing the abdominals. To do the exercise, you lie flat on your back and then lift your upper back and legs. You then push your arms up and down through the air in sets of 5 until a count of 100 is reached. This exercise not only puts a person in the *C* position (where the back is curled up) but does so under stressful circumstances.

Myth 6: An exercise mat and large ball are the two best pieces of equipment for getting a lean stomach.
An overall good diet and exercise regimen is the true key to a lean stomach. Your sneakers are actually the best piece of equipment to lose that gut. Sneakers represent fat-burning aerobic exercise. We all need to get out and walk!

Repetitive Strain Injuries

By definition, a *repetitive strain injury* is any injury that comes about after doing an action or a motion over and over again. While we generally think of repetitive strain in small joints such as the wrist or thumb, repetitive strain injuries can affect all parts of the body. The individual motion is generally simple, but the repetition of the motion compounds itself and can eventually result in intense pain. A range of repetitive motions, from small movements such as typing on a keyboard to large actions such as swinging a tennis racquet, can cause these injuries.

One of my patients is a carpenter who came to me with pain and weakness in his hands that had gotten so severe he was barely able to hold a hammer let alone swing one. After examining him, I discovered that the problem was not coming from the repetitive movements from his hands but rather the repetitive core imbalance that he developed from bending over while hammering. We treated him by correcting the core imbalance with expansion exercises; his pain diminished dramatically and quickly.

But What About My Abs?

No matter how much we teach our patients about core imbalance, many people are still looking for a great six-pack. But from the vantage point of a chiropractor, I know that a great-looking set of abdominal muscles often comes at the price of core imbalance. All those crunch exercises, sit-ups, and the Pilates Hundred emphasize tightening your body into that painful hunched-forward *C* shape, and this simply puts you in more pain.

So how do you get the six-pack abs without damaging your back and body? Here's how to build a six-pack the right way:

- Lower your percentage of body fat with aerobic exercise and proper diet.
- Use the core imbalance exercises given in this chapter.

The Best Exercises for Strong, Balanced Abdominals

The following exercises will not only fight against core imbalance but allow you to get a firm, fit stomach, too. These exercises are taught by many physical therapists and trainers, and we have selected them for you because they are the ones we find most successful in avoiding core imbalance. These exercises are easy to do, and you'll find that it will take less than 10 minutes to run through the entire program.

The anti-core-imbalance exercises are presented according to difficulty. If you aren't certain of your level, start with the beginner level, and you'll soon be able to decide how quickly you want to move to the more advanced exercises. If you increase to the maximum number of repetitions and the exercises still seem easy, then move to the next level of difficulty.

Start this program by doing one set of 12 repetitions on each side, as instructed. As you feel comfortable, increase the repetitions to a maximum of three sets of 12 repetitions.

These exercises should be performed in conjunction with an active cardio program. We recommend that our patients take a 30-minute walk four or five times a week; however, the best advice for cardio fitness is to do what you enjoy. The choice of activity—swimming, tennis, jogging, or a long walk—doesn't really matter. People who participate in a variety of activities over the course of a couple of weeks actually get the best workout. Each activity works different muscles, and that's the ideal.

Remember, too, that warming up and cooling down are important parts of any good exercise regimen. A 45-minute run should consist of a 15-minute warm-up, a 15-minute run at a rigorous but comfortable pace, and a 15-minute period during which you cool down slowly. This is the only way to safeguard your muscles.

Equipment

Most of these exercises require nothing at all. A few require the use of two different sizes of balls:

- **OVERSIZE EXERCISE BALL.** If you have room to store a big exercise ball (like the ones they have at fitness centers), you might want to purchase one. If not, do the ball-related exercise if and when you go to the gym.

- **VOLLEYBALL:** One exercise (Standing Twist with Ball) should be done with something in your hands. We usually recommend a ball the size of a volleyball, but the exercise would be equally effective if you were to hold a hardcover novel. You may also use an oversize exercise ball for this.

The Deep-Breath Test

Before starting this exercise program, take the deep-breath test. It will give you a better understand of compression and expansion.

1. Slouch in your chair. Let your arms hang down. They will naturally rotate inward. Try to take a deep breath.

2. Now sit up tall. Extend both of your arms out at your sides (like airplane wings) and take a deep breath.

3. Try it one more time, this time with your arms straight up.

As you see, you can take a much deeper breath simply by improving your posture, which in turn opens up your chest.

If breath gives us power—and it does—then think how much better you'll feel every single day if you retrain your muscles so that you can breathe deeply and easily.

You'll also find that making small changes in daily habits can lead to better breathing. Instead of reading in bed with pillows propped up behind you (with your abdomen crunched up), do your reading on the couch where your posture is more erect. Remember, too, that you should be using only one pillow when you sleep at night (see pages 77–78). The use of multiple pillows puts your spine in a C position, which reduces the amount of air you can take in.

Before and After Each Session

Complete the following steps at the beginning and end of each session:

1. Perform the Core Imbalance Test (page 100). By doing this at the beginning and end of each session, you will be able to check for core imbalance and muscle tightness. This test will remind you to stretch and relax those muscles regularly.

2. Do the Standing Abdominal Stretch before and after you exercise to fully stretch the abdominal muscles. It's also great to do when you have time throughout the day.

Do You Have Core Imbalance?
Take the Core Imbalance Test

Sit in an ordinary chair, facing forward, with your feet on the floor. Now turn your head to the right and note how far you can see behind you.

Turn back to your starting position and lift your right arm to the side. Now turn your head to the right again.

If you can see farther with your arm raised, then you have a core that is out of balance.

Standing Abdominal Stretch

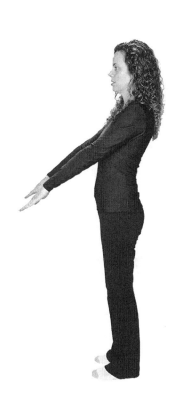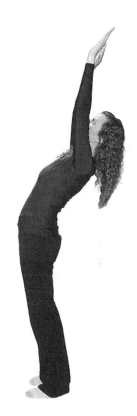

- Stand with feet about hip distance apart, knees slightly bent.
- Lift arms in front of you until they are extended straight overhead.
- Bend back slightly, stretching the abdominals.
- Repeat 12 times.

Anti-Core-Imbalance Exercises: Beginning Level

The Skinnies

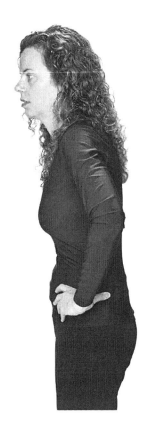 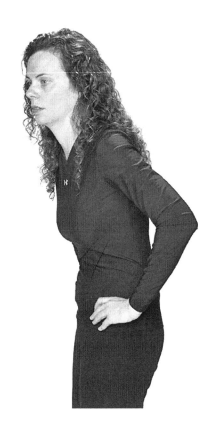

This exercise works the transverse abdominus.

- Stand, sit, or lie down on your back and exhale completely.
- Pull your navel in and up.
- Hold for 10 seconds and release.
- Repeat 12 times.

Standing Side Twist

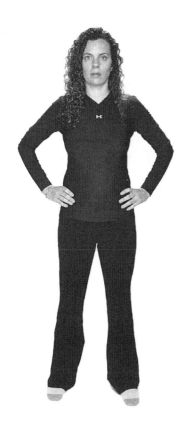 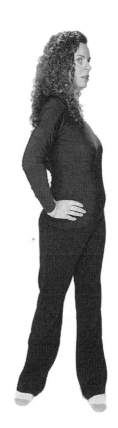

This exercise works the oblique muscles.

- Stand with hands on hips.
- With feet stationery, twist the abdomen to one side and hold for 5 seconds.
- Twist body to the other side.
- Repeat 12 times.

Ball Roll Out

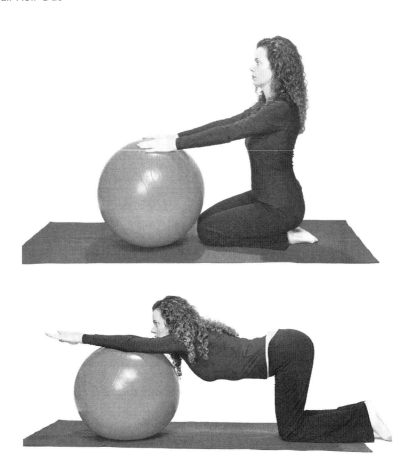

This exercise works the rectus abdominus.

- Kneel in front of an oversize exercise ball.

- Put your forearms on top of the ball and slowly roll it away from you, stretching and expanding your abdominal muscles as the ball rolls out.

- Roll the ball back in with your arms in the same position.

- Repeat 12 times.

Tummy Tucks

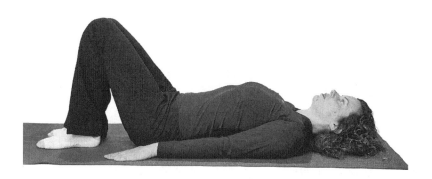

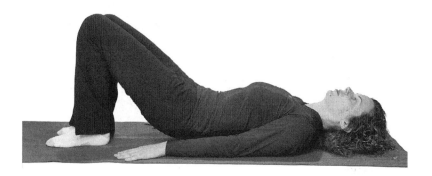

This exercise works both the transverse and the rectus abdominus.

- Lie on your back with your arms at your sides and your palms facing down.

- Draw the navel in and down toward the floor.

- Tilt your pelvis so your buttocks lift slightly off the floor.

- Hold for 10 seconds and release.

- Repeat 12 times.

Anti-Core-Imbalance Exercises: Intermediate Level

Alternate Knee Tucks

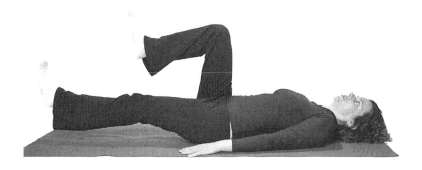

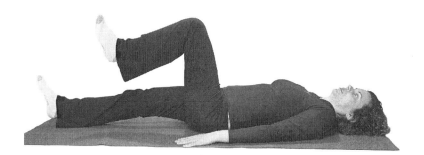

This exercise works the rectus abdominus.

- Lie on your back with your arms at your sides, your palms facing down, and your legs lying flat.
- Bend the right knee, bringing it toward your chest.
- Straighten the right knee, lowering it as you bring the left knee to your chest. (The motion resembles pedaling a bicycle.)
- Repeat 12 times.

Side Leg Raise

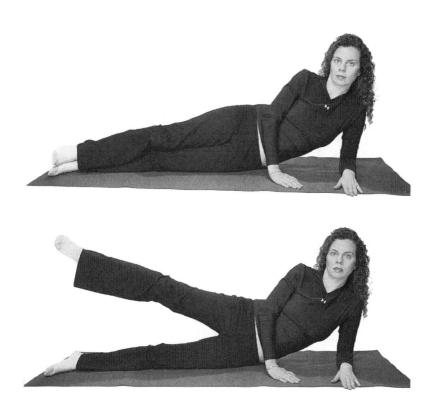

This exercise works the oblique muscles.

- Lie on the floor on your side. Bend the arm beneath you and use it to support yourself with your torso lifted to a 45-degree angle.

- Engage the side abdominals and lift the upper leg as far as you can but no further than 90 degrees.

- Repeat 12 times.

- Roll to your other side and repeat.

5-Second Plank

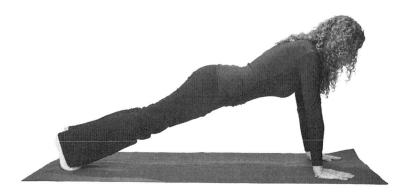

This exercise works both the rectus and transverse abdominus, building strength without the sense of failure many people experience when trying to do push-ups.

- Assume the basic push-up position: Your hands should be flat on the floor directly under the shoulders, and your body should be raised and in a straight line.

- Pull the navel in toward the spine.

- Hold for 5 seconds.

- Fully release and relax onto the floor.

- Repeat 12 times.

Standing Twist with Ball (or Book)

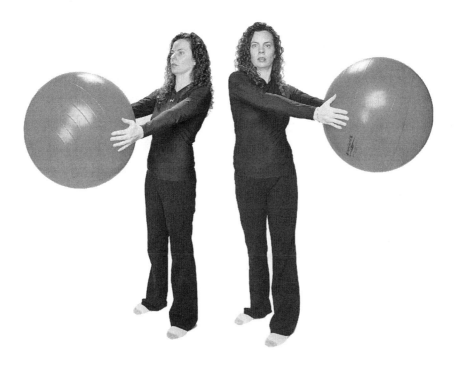

This exercise works the oblique muscles. Requires something to hold, such as an oversize exercise ball, volleyball, hardcover book, or 12-ounce water bottle.

- Stand with feet parallel, slightly apart.
- Extend your arms straight in front of you, both hands holding the object out in front of your chest.
- Twist your upper abdomen to one side.
- Hold 10 seconds.
- Twist to the other side.
- Repeat 12 times.

Anti-Core-Imbalance Exercises: Advanced Level

Single Leg Raise

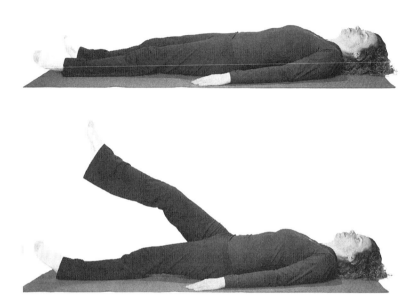

This exercise works the rectus abdominus.

- Lie on your back with your arms at your sides, your palms facing down, and your legs lying flat.

- Engage the abdominals and lift one leg off the ground at approximately a 45-degree angle.

- Slowly lower the leg.

- Repeat on the other side.

- Repeat 12 times.

Double Leg Raise

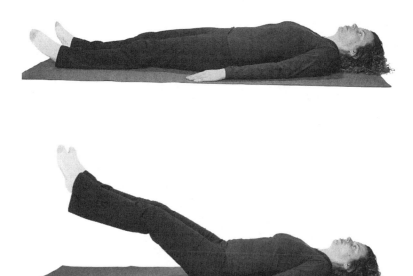

This exercise works the rectus abdominus.

- Lie on your back with your arms at your sides, your palms facing down, and your legs lying flat.

- Engage the abdominals and lift both legs slowly off the ground until they are at approximately a 45-degree angle. If this is challenging for you, put your hands under your lower back for support.

- Slowly lower both legs to the floor.

- Repeat 12 times.

Ball Lift

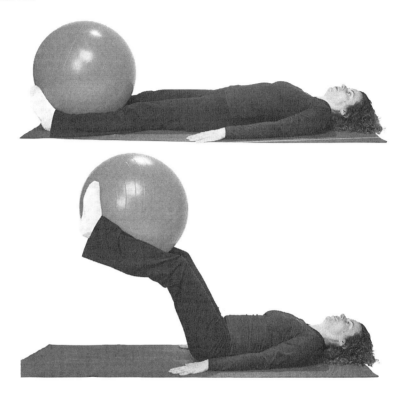

This exercise works the rectus abdominus. Requires a ball or a small pillow (something that won't hurt if you drop it).

- Lie on your back with your arms at your sides, your palms facing down, and your legs lying flat.

- Place the object between your feet.

- Lift legs slowly (no higher than 90 degrees) while your feet continue to hold the object.

- Slowly lower both legs to the floor.

- Repeat 12 times.

10-Second Plank with Leg Lift

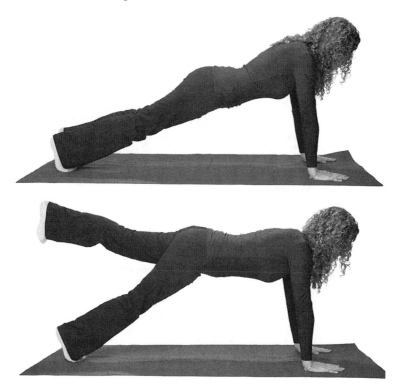

This exercise works the rectus abdominus.

- Assume the basic push-up position: Your hands should be flat on the floor directly under the shoulders, and your body should be raised and in a straight line.

- Pull the navel toward the spine.

- Lift one leg straight up behind you.

- Hold for 10 seconds.

- Repeat with the other leg.

- Repeat 12 times.

Elbow Side Plank

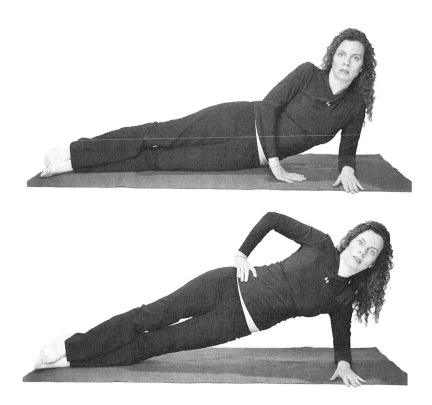

This exercise works the oblique muscles.

- Lie on your side, supporting your upper body on your forearm.
- Engage the side abdominals and lift hips toward the ceiling. (This is a side plank position: balance on the side of one foot and the forearm of that same side.)
- Hold for 10 seconds.
- Repeat 12 times.
- Roll to your other side and repeat.

PART THREE

You Are What You Eat: Body Chemistry and Back Pain

Nutrition, Digestion, and Hormones

Let food be thy medicine.

—Hippocrates

As you know from reading Chapter 1, one of the most important messages in this book is that back pain can be caused by a chemical imbalance. My father's story, related in the introduction of the book, describes the symptoms that can result from chemical imbalance as well as its possible causes. At our office, we have also treated people who suffer from back pain because they drink too much coffee, indulge in too much alcohol, or consume too many products with sugar. Some even have pain from eating too much salad!

Sugar, caffeine, too much roughage, and many other eating-related issues fall into two separate categories when it comes to determining a chemical cause for back pain:

1. **NUTRITION.** What we eat really does directly affect how we feel. For instance, sugar may give us a quick boost of energy, but we need more substantial nutrition to get us through the day.

2. **DIGESTION**. Too much roughage or certain other foods may simply be hard for your body to digest. Instead of getting a stomachache (a bodily disturbance you might expect), you may experience back pain.

This chapter also addresses hormonal causes of back pain. Most women will tell you that they are more likely to suffer aches and pains at specific points in their menstrual cycle. Studies also show that birth control pills and hormone-replacement therapy (HRT) can have a similar effect, and you'll read more about this later.

Even if your back pain is severe, don't discount a chemical cause. Pain caused by chemical issues does not present itself in a unique way; it just has distinctive causes. However, chemically induced back pain will often come and go as your diet changes or as your hormonal system fluctuates. For this reason, chemically induced back pain is particularly hard to diagnose.

Before undergoing any aggressive treatments for your back, try the chemical approach advocated in this book. Changing your diet a bit is simple—it's gentle, it's healthful, and it's noninvasive. Don't undergo unnecessary treatments when the answer may be right there on your plate.

The Case for Chemical Imbalance and Back Pain

In his book *Foods That Fight Pain*, Dr. Neal Barnard, president of the Physicians' Committee for Responsible Medicine, writes, "[S]urprising new evidence shows that food may well play a critical role in determining whether your back rebounds from the traumas of day to day life or succumbs to them." Studies analyzed by Barnard point to the importance of a good blood supply to the back to bring vital oxygen and nutrients and carry away the cells' waste products.

As we mentioned earlier, this theory is backed by a 1995 report published in the *Lancet* that described autopsies conducted by a team of researchers in Helsinki, Finland. Although the cause of death of the subjects under study had nothing to do with back pain, those who had had a history of back pain were found to have two arteries that supply the lower back completely blocked and at least one more artery severely narrowed. The study noted that people who had never reported back pain had fewer blockages. As we all know, our dietary intake is directly responsible for whether we have blocked arteries.

Although no long-term, in-depth studies have been done on general back pain and diet, we do have some data regarding specific illnesses. One of the most compelling studies comes out of the research on scoliosis, the curvature of the spine that occurs during adolescence (see page 62).

The Triad of Chemical Causes

A chemical imbalance may stem from three possible causes: nutritional factors, digestive issues, and hormonal imbalance.

Nutritional Factors

What you are eating can create toxicity within your body, which can lead to back pain. In the next chapter, we'll explore in more detail the nutritional properties of particular foods; but for our purposes here, it's important for you to know that certain foods and chemicals are inflammatory by nature.

Scientists are beginning to explore chronic inflammation as the culprit in everything from diabetes to heart disease to cancer; it's also a major player in back pain. When your spine is misaligned or your discs are squashed, the pain you feel is the result of inflammatory cells and chemicals that collect in areas of injury. Inflammatory chemicals in and around the bones and soft tissues of the back irritate nerves and send pain signals hurtling to the brain.

Other research shows that toxic environments and stressful lifestyles add to chronic inflammation. When our bodies are overloaded with toxins, our immune systems go into hyperdrive—a probable cause of chronic inflammation. When our backs are misaligned, overtaxed, or beset by a garden-variety structural problem, we are more likely to experience pain if our bodies are coping with other causes of inflammation.

But how can (fill in the blank with *salad, caffeine, cookies, spices*) be causing my back pain? If you've ever experienced an alcohol-induced hangover, you can pretty well guess how the whole thing works. Our bodies react to what we eat with a viscerosomatic response. *Viscero* means "organ"; *somatic* refers to your body, in this case the musculoskeletal system. These bodily responses occur 24 hours a day. Some of what we consume is soothing to our body; some irritates and causes pain. If you remember that a primary element of medical care often involves altering the chemical balance within your body with medications, then you'll realize that it does make sense that whatever we take in by mouth, whether it is an aspirin or an omelet, makes a difference in how we feel. This viscerosomatic response to what we eat can range from being alert after your morning caffeine to feeling sleepy from the tryptophan in turkey to getting an upset stomach from something acidic to developing back pain. Consuming a large quantity of inflammatory foods may cause your muscles to contract without relaxing. If this goes on for a prolonged period of time, back spasms and other negative health issues will result.

Cortisol, a chemical produced by the body during stressful situations, is affected by what we eat. Cortisol's job is to maintain the body's connective tissue, such as bones and muscles. "Stress hormones trigger chronic inflammation and tension in back muscles, tendons, ligaments, and discs," explains Shawn Talbot, author of *The Cortisol Connection*. And a chemical imbalance can easily trigger a cascade of stress hormones. When cortisol levels are too high, the connective tissue can become inflamed, causing pain.

Unfortunately in our high-stress culture, the body's stress response is activated so often that cortisol levels don't have a chance to return to normal, and as a result, we suffer chronic stress caused by the low-level chronic inflammation. This factor has numerous harmful health effects, and it can cause a dramatic loss of muscle tissue. When higher-than-normal levels of cortisol in the bloodstream (such as is associated with chronic stress) are prolonged, negative effects ensue, such as:

- Impaired cognitive performance

- Suppressed thyroid function

- Blood sugar imbalances, such as hyperglycemia

- Decreased bone density

- Decrease in muscle tissue

- Higher blood pressure

- Lowered immunity and inflammatory responses in the body

- Increased abdominal fat, which is associated with a greater number of health problems than fat deposited in other areas of the body. Some of the health problems associated with increased stomach fat include heart attacks, strokes, and the development of higher levels of "bad" cholesterol (LDL) and lower levels of "good" cholesterol (HDL), which can lead to other health problems.

Caffeine, alcohol, and sugars are part of many people's daily diets, and these substances have been shown to increase cortisol levels. In addition, stuffing yourself with large meals, skipping meals, or consuming only low-carbohydrate foods can result in low blood sugar, and all these situations are stressful for the body. Chronically elevated cortisol levels also increase your appetite and cravings for calorie-dense sweets and salty snacks, so the negative cycle continues. All of these factors can ultimately trigger an inflammatory reaction that results in back pain.

As you'll read in Chapter 8, some foods are known to be inflammatory and other foods are anti-inflammatory. Eating right counteracts the inflammatory cortisol process in the body.

Digestive Issues

Digestion is often closely related to nutrition, but even the person who is eating healthily may have bouts of diarrhea or constipation, which may also present as chemically caused back pain. (This may even be evident in those who take laxatives just to get their system going.) Envision your digestive system as pipes that carry out your junk. If these pipes are not working properly, waste builds up and causes pain.

Good digestion has a great deal to do with *transit time* (the time it takes for your food to pass through your body). Each type of food has a different transit time. For example, fruits are known to pass through the body quickly, but a heavy Thanksgiving dinner will have a slower transit time, or take longer to digest. If the transit times are too quick, you'll experience diarrhea; if too slow, you'll be constipated. When your body doesn't have time to absorb the proper nutrients from your food or when waste materials spend too long in your system, your health is negatively affected. For example, think of a time when you consumed a "questionable" food item in the middle of the day but your digestive system protested late in the evening. The transit time through your system determines when you suffer food-induced sickness.

When it comes to chemical balance, you want a transit time that is not too fast and not too slow, but one that is just right. Your body needs enough time to digest and absorb the nutrients from foods, and then rid the body of the waste products. An imbalanced transit time can easily create a chemical back problem. In this case, you are what you *absorb* as well as what you eat.

John, a 28-year-old marathon runner, came to our office suffering from back pain. He'd been seen by an orthopedist, who ordered a diagnostic ultrasound that failed to find the cause of his pain. The orthopedist concluded that John's pain resulted from the nonstop pounding caused by running, but John was not satisfied. As I examined John, his entire spine and body were as tight as a drum, and he talked of how tight his hamstrings were. Stretching every day for the next 10 years would never have gotten him loose. I asked all of the questions that I normally ask a patient. Once I got to the questions about his stomach and digestive functions, I became more certain about the diagnosis. John admitted that he'd been suffering from gastroesophageal reflux disease (GERD) for the last 10 years. He had tried over-the-counter remedies but for 5 years had been taking the prescription medicine Prilosec, although he hadn't seen much benefit. It was my belief that John would never get better without successfully addressing his digestive issues, and I referred him to a nutritionist.

The nutritionist identified that John's good intentions—consuming a protein drink before his morning run, drinking a sports drink, and eating sports bars as part of his daily diet—were misguided. She pointed out that regular, balanced meals are very important to all of us, particularly to an athlete. Although the types of nutritional substitutes John had been ingesting can be helpful when used occasionally, what John really needed to do was focus on eating healthy, "real" food. Now, with a new nutritional regimen, John is making great progress and suffering no pain.

Hormone Imbalance

Of course both men and women have hormones, but the issues involving hormones that cause back pain primarily affect women.

Hormonal imbalance is a major contributor to undiagnosed and unresolved back pain. Most women know that mild to uncomfortable back pain frequently accompanies menstrual bleeding—before, during, or after. A woman's monthly period should not mean a regular date with back pain, so speak with your gynecologist, endocrinologist, neuropathologist, or nutritionist about ways to create a better balance in your hormonal system so that you needn't suffer back pain.

Earlier in the book, I talked about Swedish studies that showed that women on birth control pills or hormone-replacement therapy (HRT) are more likely to suffer back pain than those who are not taking any hormonal supplements.

Pregnancy is another time when the stage is set for chemically based (hormonal) back pain. As many as 50 percent of all women experience back pain during pregnancy—even during the first trimester, before much weight gain occurs. Hormones released during pregnancy allow the ligaments in the pelvic area to soften and the joints to become looser in preparation for giving birth; this affects the mother-to-be's back. But with proper nutrition and exercise, there is no reason why this type of back pain should last beyond the birth of the baby.

Looking at Your Own Situation

There are some simple patterns that point to chemical imbalance as a cause of back pain.

To find the underlying chemical cause of pain, the first step is to determine whether there have been changes in your eating pattern that would alter the chemical system, or whether you have developed repetitive eating pattern that have become toxic and, over time, break down the body's natural resistance, or whether you are eating too much of a "good thing," such as roughage.

Getting to the root cause may be as simple as responding to the following questions, many of which you will have already addressed in the personal assessment section in Chapter 3 but are well worth reiterating here. These questions may reveal eating patterns or hormonal issues that are affecting your overall health and your back pain.

- ❑ Have you been constipated recently?

- ❑ Have you had diarrhea recently?

- ❑ Has your stomach been bothering you?

- ❑ Have you had an increase in gas?

- ❑ Have you eaten any types of food that you don't normally consume?

- ❑ Do you repetitively eat the same foods?

- ❑ Have you eaten spicy foods recently?

- ❑ Have you recently had a stomach virus?

- ❑ Have you been on any new medications?

- ❑ Have you changed your diet?

- ❑ Have you changed your vitamin regimen?

- ❑ Do you take antacids?

- ❑ Have you increased your fiber intake?

- ❑ Have you recently started to drink something different?

- ❑ Did you recently have abnormal amounts of alcohol?

- ❑ Do you drink a good deal of coffee or soda?

- ❑ Do you eat foods that are high in sugar?

- ❑ Do you use an artificial sweetener? If so, which one?

- ❑ Did you just get your menstrual period?

- ❑ Has your hormonal system undergone any recent changes (menopause, change in birth control, missed menstrual period, etc.)?

Smoking: Even Your Spine Objects

A smoker's risk of back pain is 1.5 to 2.5 times greater than that of a non-smoker. Nicotine may impair the availability of nutrients to the discs, making them more susceptible to injury. Tobacco has been shown to elevate cortisol levels and increase inflammation, which increases pain. Studies firmly show that smokers with back pain have more severe symptoms that last longer than do nonsmokers. They also have poorer outcomes after spinal surgery.

Although researchers surmise that part of the difference is that smoking dries out the spinal discs, I would add the fact that smoking also creates a chemical toxicity within the body. What you eat, drink, and smoke all affect your back.

You will want to think about your pain pattern. Sometimes it is easy to trace your pain to poor dietary choices that also resulted in reflux, gas pains, diarrhea, or constipation.

The Good News

The good news about chemical-induced back pain is that it is the easiest type of back pain to fix. You don't have to do extra exercises, no one is going to order you to relax, and there's no discussion of surgery. All you have to do is learn what foods are causing you distress. Proper foods can be the best medicine that you can ever have. The anti-back-pain diet, which is outlined in Chapter 9, has saved countless people from undergoing radical treatment and unnecessary back surgeries that would have been unsuccessful.

So what do you have to lose? Could the cause of your back problem be a chemical imbalance? Is this the missing link in solving your particular back problem? If you've tried other solutions without results, and the self-diagnosis questions in Chapter 3 have pointed toward a possible chemical imbalance, then my strong recommendation is that you take a fresh look at your dietary intake. With appropriate treatment, you should notice a difference within 3 to 4 weeks. If changing your diet or making other lifestyle choices to remedy the chemical imbalances in your body doesn't resolve the immediate problem, at least you will not have spent a lot of money on doctor bills. But you may have adopted healthier eating habits for 4 weeks, which will likely give you more energy and maybe help you drop a few extra pounds. Either way, you win.

Chapter 8 outlines some general information on what you need to know about various foods. Chapter 9 provides actual diet plans for you to follow.

Food Rules for
Healthy Backs

One Saturday afternoon I received a phone call from a Grammy-winning recording artist who was suffering from severe upper back and neck pain and was concerned that she was not going to be able to make it through her performance on *Saturday Night Live* and a concert that was scheduled for the following day. She said the pain was so bad she could barely turn her head.

During the examination, I noticed that her whole muscular system was tight, almost to the point of rigidity. It was as if she were suffering from a full-body spasm. From the examination, which includes an assessment of the abdominal area, I could tell that she was suffering severe gas pains. We talked for a while, and she told me about her on-the-road diet, which was not very healthy and frequently featured tasty treats like toaster pastries and ice cream. It became clear to me that her primary problem—so serious that it caused back and neck tension and pain—stemmed from bad eating.

I presented her with the good news. I explained that I understood how very uncomfortable she was (and how very real her pain was) and that although I couldn't cure her immediately, I knew she could feel much better within a few days. (When the physical reaction is this severe, it reflects a toxic buildup within the body, which requires a reorientation of the diet and time for the body to readjust.)

Bad Habits Compound Other Problems

Like the Grammy winner I just described, most of my patients say they don't have much time to prepare meals. When asked to keep a food diary, which I ask of most of my patients, a typical day's entry will read like this:

BREAKFAST: coffee, muffin or bagel, more coffee

LUNCH: sandwich, chips, soda or iced tea

SNACK: candy or chips, more soda

DINNER: pizza or pasta dish, soda or wine, pastry or ice cream

Does this list look familiar? It's pretty clear that this kind of eating doesn't provide you with nearly the vitamins and nutrients you need to stay healthy.

If you put low-performance fuel into what needs to be your high-performance body, there is little surprise that your back and body aren't functioning at their peak. If you are concerned about your health, you need to upgrade the fuel you consume. But even people who place great value on exercising and eating right can run into trouble if the balance of food is incorrect, causing pain-related issues.

Too Much of a Good Thing

Curiously, those patients (about 20 percent) whose back pain has been clearly linked to chemical or nutritional factors ate healthily. But many had very little variety in their diets. These people were actually eating too much of a good thing. Keeping a food diary was easy for them because they ate almost the exact same thing every day. Unfortunately, this system doesn't work. Your body needs multiple sources of the vitamins, minerals, and other nutrients it needs. Ironically, when it comes to food choices, a certain level of inconsistency is ideal. Because these patients didn't eat a variety of healthy food, their dietary systems were constantly irritated. Many of these patients had gassiness, a bloated feeling, abdominal pain, diarrhea, and even constipation. In these cases, we strive to get the patients eating a more balanced diet. Over time their digestive systems slow down, and the transit time becomes more accommodating for positive absorption—and their back pain goes away.

Before I understood this, I went on my own health kick. I started having oatmeal—which is high in fiber—every day for breakfast, and salads were my choice for lunch. Unfortunately, a week into this diet, I had a dramatic increase in bloating and stomach pain—and eventually a stiff neck. When I returned to my old eating habits, which were already pretty good, I felt better. The moral of the story is that just because a food is considered healthful doesn't mean it is always good for you—or acceptable to eat in excess.

So what healthy foods cause trouble? The most frequent offenders include salad, oatmeal, egg whites, tofu, smoothies, raw vegetables, frozen yogurt, beans, freshly squeezed juices, and protein bars. The demon in many cases is often too much roughage. Although we all need some roughage for proper digestion, too much causes your digestive tract to go into overdrive.

One patient, Paul, offers a good example of what can happen with too much of a good thing. Although he was trying to adjust his lifestyle for better health, he found that the process could be painful. Recently he came to me complaining of lower back pain that was so severe he couldn't lift or play with his 1-year-old twins. He had been following my stretching regimen before and after he exercised, and he was quite miffed to be suffering from debilitating pain.

When I asked him to explain what had happened, he said he "just kind of woke up with the pain" after playing basketball the day before. He had no recollection of getting injured, but he surmised he was just getting too old to play, joking that he was worried his illustrious career was over at the age of 35.

I went through my regular questions. He had just told me about his exercise and stretching routine, so I continued: Had he been stressed? No. Had he eaten anything different? No. But then he paused. He mentioned he had just gotten back from a spa where they talked about the benefit of flaxseed oil, so he had begun to put flaxseeds on all of his food.

As I continued this line of questioning, it became clear that the flaxseeds created too much irritation to Paul's digestive system and, in turn, caused muscle inflammation, which resulted in severe back spasms.

I suggested that he stop eating the flaxseeds and reduce the amount of roughage in his diet for a time to let his system calm down. He was pain-free within a week.

Quick Tips for Eating Well

- Eat something within 1 hour of getting up each morning.

- Have at least one healthful snack between meals each day.

- Eat slowly to allow yourself to be aware of feeling full.

- Avoid the clean-plate club. Always leave at least one bite of each type of food on your plate at the end of the meal.

- Keep a food journal for at least 1 week, maybe longer.

The Food Diary

At the outset of treatment, every patient is encouraged to keep track of what he or she eats—and when—for 1 week. We also ask them to take note of any special circumstance that might affect their eating patterns, such as travel, illness, or special events. We don't recommend that they modify what they eat because the purpose of this written record is to evaluate their *normal* eating and drinking patterns, so we can look for the usual suspects: too many sweets (particularly unrefined sugars), processed foods, caffeine, and alcohol. We also check to see if the patient is skipping meals, going a long time between eating, eating too much, or eating too little.

Events such as travel can really throw a person's digestive system off track. Waiting too long between meals can also make a big difference in how you feel as well as contribute to a habit of binge eating.

Food Rules

Over time, we formulated seven general rules to help our patients create a healthy diet.

Rule 1: Watch your weight.

Being overweight is actually a contributing factor to structural imbalance; the more weight your bones must bear, the more difficulty your spine has in bearing that weight properly. However, there is a reason we chose to address this issue in the chemical section of the book rather than in the structural part of this book. Although excess weight can certainly contribute to structural back pain, we have come to believe that excess weight is a greater factor in back problems because of the chemical toxicity and unhealthy eating habits. In essence, people who are overweight are not following healthy eating patterns. The unhealthy habits are the cause of chemical back pain; the weight is an additional unfortunate effect.

Rule 2: Drink plenty of water.

Many of my patients simply don't drink enough water. They come in with a cup of flavored coffee from the corner coffee shop and think that the bottled iced tea they have with lunch and the beer they order with dinner constitute fluid. But these other liquids are not the same as water.

We all need to drink water. Drinking enough water actually helps with back pain. Lack of water causes the area around the spinal discs to become dry, and little fissures (cracks) can form. If the fissures become severe, then the inside of the disc can bulge and put pressure on your spinal nerves or spinal cord—a very painful condition.

Rule 3: Take a multivitamin.

An exciting study published in the *Journal of Nutrition* revealed that taking a multivitamin actually reduces the risk of heart attacks. Women and men who took a multivitamin supplement suffered 33 percent and 22 percent fewer heart attacks, respectively, than women and men who did not take a supplement. When choosing a multivitamin and mineral supplement, remember that it is meant to do what its name implies: *supplement*—not replace—a healthful diet. People prone to back problems should take vitamins and minerals that strengthen bones and cartilage, such as calcium, magnesium, vitamins C and D, and manganese. In addition, various other supplements are worth trying, either singly or in combination. Consult with a nutritionist or medical professional to decide what and how much to take.

Here are some guidelines for buying vitamins and other supplements:

- **VITAMINS.** For most vitamins, a supplement should provide no more than 100 percent of the daily recommended value. You want at least 100 percent of the daily value of vitamins D, B_1 (thiamin), B_2 (riboflavin), B_3 (niacin), B_6, and B_{12} and folic acid. Look for at least 20 micrograms of vitamin K. At least 40 percent of the vitamin A should be in the form of beta-carotene.

- **MINERALS.** Look for a supplement with up to 100 percent of the daily value of copper, zinc, and iodine. You want no more than 200 micrograms of selenium and chromium. Calcium is a very large mineral and takes up so much space in a multivitamin supplement that it is difficult to include 100 percent of the daily value in one capsule. An additional calcium supplement (containing vitamin D) is usually needed.

- **NIACINAMIDE.** This form of niacin, a B vitamin, may be effective against arthritic back pain; try for 500 milligrams three times a day. This B vitamin has also been helpful in reducing the symptoms of carpal tunnel syndrome.

- **USP.** Look for the letters *USP*—which stand for United States Pharmacopeia—on the label. This means the brand of multivitamin

Got Calcium?

Calcium is an important mineral, which helps us fight off arthritis and osteoarthritis, both of which can cause debilitating pain and suffering. When it comes to calcium, the key point is not just the amount of calcium that you consume (or take in supplement form) but the amount that your body is able to absorb. To properly absorb calcium, your body must have enough vitamin D, which can be gained through sun exposure or supplementation.

In 1993, a group of Yale University researchers studied the occurrence of hip fractures in 16 countries. The scientists expected to find that the countries with the greatest calcium consumption would have the fewest hip fractures, but the opposite was true. Countries with high calcium consumption actually had more hip fractures. The researchers noted that the greatest number of fractures were in countries with high consumption of processed foods. These processed foods interfere with calcium absorption.

Also, caffeine, alcohol, sodium, and tobacco are also known to deplete calcium from the body. A lifestyle and diet high in these substances dramatically increases your chance for hip fractures.

has been tested to ensure that the levels of nutrients listed on the label are the levels that are actually in the product.

- **EXPIRATION DATE.** Note how many capsules you need to take each day. Is it feasible to use the entire container before the expiration date? If not, consider buying a smaller amount.

The body's nutrient needs change as it goes through different life-cycle stages. Choosing an appropriate group-specific multivitamin (such as a children's, women's, or men's formula) can provide the right combination of nutrients you need without anything you don't.

Rule 4: Cut down on caffeine.

Caffeine has been proven to increase muscle contractions. Taking in large or regular doses of caffeine can lead to muscle spasms and cramping. These factors can certainly be part of the cause of your back pain.

Rule 5: Reduce intake of sugars and sweeteners.

The average American drinks more than 486 sodas a year, according to the soft drink association. If you calculate that an average sugared soda contains 10 teaspoons of sugar—or the equivalent of artificial sweetener—you begin to understand that this just can't be good for your body.

For better health, cut down on all sugars and sweeteners. The average amount of sugar consumption per person each year in the United States is a shocking 175 pounds. Sugar increases the rate at which you excrete calcium—not at all good for your bones. Also stay away from artificial sweeteners, such as saccharine and aspartame, which can even be worse for you than sugar. According to the U.S. Food and Drug Administration (FDA), aspartame accounted for over 75 percent of the adverse food reactions reported to the administration before 1995, when the agency stopped accepting reports on adverse reactions to aspartame.

In a small but interesting study reported in the *American Journal of Medicine* in 1984, researchers at the Veterans Administration Medical Center in Minneapolis tested pain tolerance in eight healthy young men. They found that when they gave the men an intravenous infusion of sugar, the men's pain sensitivity increased markedly. The men were aware of the pain sooner and experienced it more intensely. The researchers then tested people with diabetes who had higher than normal blood sugars. The researchers found the same thing. The pain sensitivity of the people with diabetes was much higher than that of people with normal blood sugar levels.

Rule 6: Read food labels carefully.

Reading food labels today is as difficult as trying to remember a foreign language you studied in school years ago. The ingredients are printed in type so small that you need reading glasses to see them, and there are so many chemicals listed that it is impossible to understand what is in the food.

Check the ingredient list on your packaged foods. Look for food with few chemicals listed and be aware of the order in which the ingredients are listed. The food is primarily made up of the first four or five ingredients. The other ingredients are included in greatly reduced amounts, so they are less important.

Food Sensitivities

While food allergies used to be quite rare, medical professionals are seeing an increasing number of them. For reasons we don't yet understand, more and more people are being diagnosed with food sensitivities that cause serious pain. Whether food allergies are simply being more widely recognized by increasingly sophisticated diagnostic techniques, or whether the chemicals added to our food and the environment have made a difference, we have found a growing number of patients with back pain who also suffer from food sensitivities.

Beware of any word that ends in *-ose*. If an ingredient ends in the suffix *-ose*, it is a sugar. Sometimes the most surprising processed foods (salsa, ketchup, prepared foods) have sugar added to them.

Watch out for these other red-flag ingredients:

- **HYDROGENATED OR PARTIALLY HYDROGENATED OILS**

- **TRANS-FATS**, which are made when vegetable oils are exposed to hydrogen so that they became solid at room temperature. Trans-fats were added to foods because they lengthen shelf life; unfortunately, however, they are detrimental to our health. As a result, trans-fats are now being removed from many prepared foods.

- **INTERESTERIFIED FAT** (called *interesterified soybean* or *stated rich oil* on the label), which has been shown to lower HDL (good cholesterol), increase blood glucose levels, and depress insulin levels

- **ENRICHED WHEAT FLOUR**, which is neither whole wheat nor oat bran flour and does not deliver the nutrients and fiber you need

- **OTHER ADDITIVES**, including those that end with *-ates* or *-ites*, as in nitrates and nitrites, which are frequently found in processed meats

- **FOOD COLORING**, which is for the most part an unnatural ingredient

- **TYRAMINE**, which is a naturally occurring substance formed from the breakdown of proteins as food ages and is found in most alcoholic beverages, aged cheeses, and processed meats. Tyramine has been associated with increased systolic blood pressure and migraines.

Rule 7: Listen to your body.

If you had Chinese food last night and you don't feel well this morning, consider: Was it the three beers you had with dinner, or was it the food itself? If you routinely get a stomachache after consuming milk products, you might have lactose intolerance. Start paying attention to which foods agree with you and which ones don't, so you can avoid the ingredients that upset your system, and you'll soon find you're feeling better all around.

CHAPTER 9

The No More Back Pain Diet

The heart of this chapter is the daily eating plan that provides a detoxifying, anti-inflammatory, anti-pain diet. It is easy to follow and can be tailored to your individual needs and tastes. Commit to this plan for 4 short weeks and, like our many patients who've followed this program successfully, you, too, will readily see how it will lead to overall well-being as well as a healthier back and spine!

The No More Back Pain Diet

Your diet has a huge impact on your back pain. Muscles and organs contract and relax in the process of doing their jobs. Their motions make digestion possible, but refined carbohydrates, excess sugar, and caffeine throw our stomachs into turmoil and cause the muscles involved in digestion to contract for an extended period. The result? Spasms and pain.

One obvious example of this turmoil is a hangover. By saturating your body with alcohol, you send your muscles and organs into a state of extended contraction. It's no wonder you wake up feeling stiff, achy, and foggy headed. If you had consumed a fresh berry smoothie and some sparkling water, chances are you would not be feeling like your head had a train running through it!

Nutritional balance is a vital part of freeing yourself from, and preventing, back pain. The No More Back Pain Diet has been designed to target and eliminate certain toxins from your system. It will make a dramatic difference in how you feel and how your body will function. Adopting this diet will not only alleviate the aches and pains in your back but have a significantly positive effect on your overall health. This anti-back-pain diet addresses different levels of back pain (from mild to severe) and offers various starting points, depending on the severity of your pain.

The diet for severe back pain is for people who can barely move because their pain is so severe. If you have trouble getting out of bed and can't bend to tie your shoes, you should start with this diet, following it for 4 days or less. You will progress through the next phase over a period of 4 weeks. Those who have less severe back pain will start with the mild to moderate plan. The guidelines conclude with a long-term maintenance plan that is so easy to follow, patients don't seem to have any trouble sticking with it.

This diet is great for everyone—even those without back pain. You and your family will find that balanced and nutritious meals like these simply make you feel better.

Why the Cookbook Approach Doesn't Work

The problem with most diets is that they take a one-size-fits-all approach: Do this and you will get the results you want. A diet plan can be helpful, but there is no one approach that works for everyone. Each person has individual needs that must be met to create his or her unique chemical balance.

As you get underway with this new diet plan, listen to your body. How do you feel when following the diet? The ideal eating plan leaves you feeling satisfied and energized. If you feel gassy, bloated, or fatigued after a meal, it wasn't right for you. (Keep in mind that vitamins and medications can also create this phenomenon.) Pay attention to your body and do what is right for you.

From the lists of approved foods, select those that seem most appropriate for you and then adjust as needed.

General Guidelines

What follows is a detailed rundown of the No More Back Pain Diet as well as a list of approved and nonapproved foods. There are also sample menus to give you an overall vision of how a day of eating on the diet might look. Don't feel tied to the menus given here; these are just suggestions. Just make sure that you are eating foods that are on the approved list. And remember to drink plenty of water—try for eight 8-ounce glasses a day. You can drink flavored seltzer water, too—just make sure the only ingredients are *water* and *natural flavors.*

Approved Foods

- **WHOLE GRAINS,** including whole grain breads, whole grain pastas, whole grain cereals, whole grain tortillas, and whole grain baked goods (look for the words *whole grain* on the food label followed by the name of a grain, such as wheat, corn, rice, oats, barley, quinoa, sorghum, and rye)

- **OATMEAL OR CORNMEAL**

- **SOY FLOUR**

- **NUTS AND SEEDS,** including nut and seed oils; nut and seed butters; unsweetened coconut; vegetable oils, olive oil, and flaxseed oil

- **PROTEIN,** including chicken, fish (especially mackerel, lake trout, herring, sardines, albacore tuna, and salmon), lean cuts of meat (turkey, pork, beef), eggs, and cheese

- **VEGETABLES**—all including starchy vegetables such as sweet potatoes, potatoes, corn, butternut squash, and peas

The Value of Organic Produce

There are several benefits to organic produce (edibles grown without the use of drugs, hormones, or synthetic chemicals). One is that eating organic produce (or foods made using organic produce) limits your exposure to pesticides. Another is that organic farming practices reduce pollution and conserve water and soil—all things designed to benefit the environment. Fruits and veggies provide us with so many vital nutrients, but if you're ingesting a bunch of pesticides with your apple or broccoli, what's the use?

Most pesticide residue is left on the skin of fruits and vegetables, so it may be tempting to peel them, but the skin and just below the skin is where a lot of the nutrients are found. Buying only organic produce is one way to minimize pesticide residue dangers, but organic produce can get pretty expensive (especially if you've got a large family). The Environmental Working Group has tested the pesticide residue levels on dozens of fruits and veggies and has ranked them based on pesticide levels. These findings help us determine which produce should be eaten only if organically grown and which ones are okay to consume if commercially grown.

Always buy organic varieties of the following foods because when conventionally farmed, they have a high level of pesticide residue:

Apples	**Grapes, imported**	**Potatoes**
Bell peppers	**Nectarines**	**Raspberries**
Celery	**Peaches**	**Spinach**
Cherries	**Pears**	**Strawberries**

It is acceptable to buy these conventionally grown foods because they have minimal pesticide residues:

Asparagus	**Cauliflower**	**Papaya**
Avocados	**Kiwi**	**Pineapples**
Bananas	**Mangoes**	**Sweet corn**
Broccoli	**Onions**	**Sweet peas**

- **FRUIT**—all except those listed in the nonapproved list

- **DECAFFEINATED COFFEE/TEA** (unsweetened)

- **SELTZER WATER**—plain and flavored (look for *water* and *natural flavor* as the only ingredients)

- **WATER**

Nonapproved Foods

- **ENRICHED WHITE FLOUR**, commonly found in breads, pastas, biscuits, waffles, crackers, muffins, cereals, pancakes, croutons, rolls, pretzels, graham crackers, cookies, baked goods, and tortillas

- **HYDROGENATED OILS** (look for the words *trans-fat, partially hydrogenated oil,* and *hydrogenated oil* on the food label)*

- **CREAM CHEESE AND PROCESSED CHEESES**

- **SOME FRUITS**, such as grapes, bananas, cherries, figs, and dried fruit

- **ARTIFICIALLY FLAVORED AND/OR SWEETENED FRUIT DRINKS** *

- **GRAPE JUICE** (even unsweetened)

- **MILK SHAKES AND MALTS**

- **SOFT DRINKS**, including diet sodas*

- **MEAL-REPLACEMENT SHAKES**

- **HOT CHOCOLATE AND CHOCOLATE MILK**

- **WINE, BEER, SPIRITS, AND CORDIALS**

- **CAFFEINATED COFFEE/TEA**

- **ADDED SWEETENERS**, including sugar, molasses, honey, agave nectar, and artificial sweeteners

- **PACKAGED OR PROCESSED FOOD**—look for words ending in *-ose* on the food label

Some of the nonapproved foods can be added back to your diet once you have completed 3 to 4 weeks of Phase I of the No More Back Pain Diet. Note, however, that you should always strive to avoid ingesting the foods marked with an asterisk (*), even when you've reached the maintenance phase.

Getting Started

Plan to begin this diet on a Friday. During the weekend, people generally have the most free time to clear their schedule in case they suffer from the withdrawal symptoms of eliminating caffeine and sugar from their diets.

Shopping

Get rid of the junk food in your house and stock up on healthy food. Initially, this diet will be expensive; however, once you have the basics, healthy eating generally costs about the same as eating prepackaged junk food. (Your health is certainly worth any added cost!)

Cook Ahead

Do the majority of your cooking and prep work on the weekend. This will allow you to plan out your snacks and meals throughout the week, reducing your chances of being unprepared and not having the right foods at your disposal. Grill some chicken cutlets, boil some eggs, cut up extra vegetables to use as snacks, package up some almonds or cashews as high-energy foods to-go.

It may take you some time to get used to this new way of eating. The first week is the toughest, but it gets progressively easier from there.

Don't Let Yourself Get Hungry

The recommended portion sizes are guidelines—adjust as you need to. This is not a weight-loss diet, even though most people will lose weight. We don't want you to be hungry, but we certainly don't want you to overeat, either.

If you dislike a particular food listed on a menu, make a reasonable substitution. For example, if you don't like the taste of or don't feel well after eating eggs, simply don't eat them. The approved and nonapproved lists of food will be helpful in making selections that are right for you and your personal preferences.

Don't Do It Halfway

Try to maintain this eating plan for at least 4 weeks. Although your body will feel a difference chemically within 3 weeks, it takes longer than that to create new habits and to let your body fully adjust to this new way of eating. It also permits you to make a few missteps without driving yourself crazy. If the sauce you had at the in-laws had a little sugar in it, don't worry. Just get right back to the diet. (Too many people use diet slip-ups as deal breakers.) Just do the best you can—be kind to yourself, and maintain the majority of the principles. You'll soon be feeling better for it!

Phase I: Diet for Severe Back Pain

When you're suffering from severe back pain, your body is suffering from inflammation. Before you can begin to feel the benefits of removing toxins and irritants from your diet, you must let your muscles and digestive system calm down. The goal of this phase of the diet is to remove inflammation. (*Note:* The diet for severe back pain does not fulfill general nutritional needs, but it is designed to be used very briefly in order to calm the inflammatory response in your system.) Just as you can easily survive for a few days of only eating soup and toast during a bout with a stomach bug, you will also be fine eating only the foods on this bland diet for a few days.

Basic Action

Although it may sound counter to all the standard diet advice you've heard, we're going to ask you to remove all of the fiber, also known as roughage, from your diet. This means no whole grains, nuts, or raw fruits and vegetables (you may eat them well-cooked, though). You must remove chips (all types), all spicy foods, caffeine, and alcohol. Think of this as the sort of diet you eat when you are fighting off a bad cold or soothing a stomachache. Some people call it a bland diet, but we prefer to think of it as the *clean slate phase.* You'll be creating an environment in your body that is very calm, soothing, and receptive to the healthful and nutritious changes you'll make in the No More Back Pain Diet.

You are probably thinking that it is counterintuitive to eat fewer fruits and vegetables and complex carbohydrates when you have severe back pain. You are right. But we do not consider this a long-term way to eat.

Complex carbohydrates, which include most fruits and vegetables, comprise vitamins, minerals, and fiber. Because they are multidimensional, they need a well-functioning digestive system to process. Simply put, roughage can be rough to digest. On the other hand, simple carbohydrate foods are limited in nutritional content and virtually fiber-free. Though simple carbs are missing many good things, foods like white rice and white bread offer the benefit of being easy to digest.

For the severe back pain sufferer, the simple foods that the body can process easily give the irritated digestive system a time-out to heal. Once the digestive system has calmed down—after about 4 days—we recommend returning to the whole grain foods that are the basis of the moderate recommendations of the diet.

Duration

Follow this phase of the diet for a *maximum* of 4 days. Even 1 or 2 days may be enough for people who don't usually drink caffeine or alcohol. If you normally consume caffeine or alcohol on a daily basis, then follow this phase for 3 or 4 days.

What to Expect

Though the bland diet might seem a little boring, you'll be following these guidelines only briefly, and they should help your digestive system calm down. If you're a committed coffee drinker, you will probably go through caffeine withdrawal during this step. You may experience headaches or even flu-like symptoms. (The duration of the withdrawal symptoms varies from person to person, but symptoms generally do not last for more than a week.) If you're accustomed to high-fiber cereal, fruits, and vegetables, you may feel deprived and could experience mild constipation. Remember, this phase lasts a maximum of 4 days; after you've completed this step, you'll move on to Phase II and then you'll really begin to feel the back pain relief!

Sample Meals

DAY 1

Breakfast
4 ounces fruit juice (not grape)
1 bowl of puffed rice cereal with skim milk or soy milk
6 ounces plain or low-fat yogurt with cinnamon
1 cup decaffeinated herbal tea

Lunch
1 grilled cheese sandwich on white bread
1 bowl of chicken noodle soup

Dinner
Mixed steamed veggies with a small amount of butter or margarine
1 grilled or broiled filet mignon
1 baked potato without skin, topped with plain yogurt and chives

DAY 2

Breakfast
4 ounces fruit juice (not grape)
2 scrambled eggs
2 pieces white toast with butter
1 cup decaffeinated herbal tea

Lunch
1 grilled chicken breast on a roll with light mayonnaise

Dinner
Roast chicken
Roasted potatoes
Well-cooked peas, broccoli, or green beans

DAY 3

Breakfast
4 ounces fruit juice (not grape)
1 frozen waffle (not whole wheat), topped with butter or plain or vanilla yogurt
1 cup decaffeinated herbal tea

Lunch
  1 baked potato with sour cream

Dinner
  1 bowl chicken soup with white rice

DAY 4

Breakfast
  4 ounces fruit juice (not grape)

  1 plain bagel with butter

  1 cup decaffeinated herbal tea

Lunch
  1 turkey sandwich on white bread with light mayonnaise and mustard

Dinner
  1 bowl of pasta (not whole wheat) tossed with olive oil

  Well-cooked vegetables

Daily Snacks
  Graham or plain crackers

  White bread or rolls

  Pretzels

  Plain or vanilla yogurt

Phase II: Diet for Mild to Moderate Back Pain

Think of this as the beginning of the healthiest time of your life! For the next 3 to 4 weeks, you will be eating the optimal diet to eliminate toxic buildup and bring your body back to its natural balance. If you were experiencing severe back pain, this will be Phase II for you. You've eliminated certain foods from your diet and are now ready to reintroduce the most healthful foods.

In this phase, as you eliminate the toxic foods you will be creating lasting balance that will result in increased energy, better resistance to illness, greater mental ability, and reduced aches and pains.

Basic Action

Though the diet for severe back pain removed all roughage from the diet, the emphasis in this phase of the diet is to eat healthily. The meal plans reflect both quantity and quality. Processed carbohydrates, added sugars, and caffeine react toxically and create an environment of inflammation and turmoil inside your body. Eliminating these foods brings your body back to balance and allows it to focus on doing everything it was designed to do—like digesting food, pumping blood, thinking, and moving. But just as important as eating healthy food is eating healthy *amounts* of food. Remember, eating excessive amounts of even the most healthful foods creates a toxic environment in your body and leads to structural problems, discomfort, and pain.

In general, I hesitate to recommend a number of portions or to give you fixed amounts of specific foods because everybody is different. It's important for you to eat until you're satisfied but *never* until you're full. Think simple—choose whole grains; lean, fresh proteins; and real food that is as close to nature as possible. Refer to the lists of approved and nonapproved foods and the sample menus to guide you through your food choices. The only beverages allowed are water, flavored seltzer water (as long as the only two ingredients are water and natural flavors), and decaffeinated/herbal tea.

Duration

Stay on this plan for 3 to 4 weeks.

What to Expect

Your first week on the No More Back Pain Diet may be a challenge, especially if your body currently relies on the sugar rushes and nervous energy buzzes caused by refined carbohydrates, added sugars, and caffeine. If you're coming into this stage after following the recommendations for severe back pain, then you've already cut out caffeine and may already be past any withdrawal symptoms. If not, expect mild flu-like symptoms and headaches for up to 1 week after removing caffeine from your diet. Sounds pretty unpleasant, but I guarantee it will be well worth it.

After the first 2 weeks, you will begin to feel the intense benefits of the diet.

Your body will feel less stiff, more limber. You'll feel clear headed and have enough energy to take on each day. You'll feel more in control.

Sample Meals

DAY 1

Breakfast
> 1 egg plus 2 egg whites, scrambled in 1 teaspoon olive oil
>
> 1 slice whole grain toast with ½ teaspoon butter
>
> ½ grapefruit

Lunch
> 1 medium-size tossed salad (veggies only, no croutons or cheese) topped with grilled chicken or tuna (no mayonnaise)
>
> 2 tablespoons oil and vinegar dressing

Dinner
> 1 bowl of whole grain pasta tossed with 1 tablespoon olive oil and crushed fresh garlic to taste
>
> Grilled or steamed mixed vegetables with white beans

Snack
> ½ cup mixed berries with 1 tablespoon crushed walnuts

DAY 2

Breakfast
> 1 cup low-fat plain yogurt
>
> ¼ cantaloupe
>
> 1 slice whole grain toast with 1 teaspoon nut butter

Lunch
> 1 slice whole grain bread topped with sliced turkey breast, lettuce, tomato, and 1 teaspoon light mayonnaise
>
> 1 cup low-fat cottage cheese

Dinner
> 3 to 4 ounces lean steak, grilled or broiled
>
> 1 small side salad (veggies only) with balsamic vinegar
>
> ½ baked sweet potato (can substitute white potato)
>
> Steamed broccoli or mixed vegetables

Snack

½ cup unsweetened applesauce mixed with ¼ cup whole grain cereal, sprinkled with cinnamon

DAY 3

Breakfast

1 cup plain cooked oats (old-fashioned rolled or quick) with ½ cup diced apple and 1 tablespoon crushed walnuts, sprinkled with cinnamon

Lunch

Mixed greens with assorted veggies, topped with lean turkey, ham, and natural cheese and drizzled with 2 tablespoons oil and vinegar dressing

1 very small whole grain roll or 1 slice whole grain bread

Dinner

1 broiled chicken breast, seasoned with lemon, garlic, onions, and parsley

Mixed vegetables (roasted with 1 tablespoon olive oil)

½ cup brown rice or quinoa

Snack

½ cup pineapple (fresh or canned in own juice) with a dollop of low-fat plain yogurt, sprinkled with 1 teaspoon crushed walnuts

DAY 4

Breakfast

1 whole grain English muffin topped with 1 poached egg, 1 slice Canadian bacon or lean turkey, and sliced tomato

Apple, sliced and sprinkled with cinnamon

Lunch

Roasted vegetable sandwich made with ½ cup roasted mixed veggies and 1 slice cheese, on 2 slices whole grain bread spread with hummus

Dinner

6 ounces lean ground turkey or beef (at least 94 percent lean) mixed with unsweetened tomato sauce and veggies (onions, peppers, and mushrooms)

1 bowl of whole wheat or brown rice pasta

Snack
½ cup unsweetened granola

DAY 5

Breakfast
Oatmeal with 2 tablespoons chopped walnuts and sliced pear, sprinkled with cinnamon

½ cup skim or unsweetened soy milk

Lunch
Chef's salad made with mixed greens, turkey, ham, cheese, and raw vegetables, dressed with oil and vinegar dressing

Whole wheat English muffin with hummus

Dinner
Roasted pork tenderloin

Baked sweet potato topped with cinnamon and dollop of plain yogurt

Broccoli sautéed in garlic and olive oil

Snack
Unsweetened applesauce, sprinkled with cinnamon

DAY 6

Breakfast
1 whole wheat bagel or 1 slice whole grain bread

1 tablespoon almond butter

6 ounces plain nonfat yogurt with ½ cup mixed frozen organic berries, sprinkled with cinnamon

Lunch
Cooked lentils mixed with quinoa, spinach, and crushed peanuts

Seasoned grilled tofu

1 bowl vegetable soup

Dinner
1 poached chicken breast

Brown rice

Roasted root vegetables

DAY 7

Breakfast

Oat bran flakes mixed with puffed wheat cereal

½ cup skim or soy milk

½ cup strawberries

2 tablespoons raw almonds

Lunch

Avocado and black bean roll-up made with 1 oat bran tortilla spread with thin layer of no-fat yogurt, avocado, black beans, salsa, and brown rice

Add grilled chicken or tofu, if desired

Dinner

1 bowl of vegetable soup made with low-sodium stock (vegetable or chicken) and fresh or frozen vegetables

6 ounces grilled lamb chop

Spinach and garlic, stir-fried in 1 tablespoon olive oil

½ cup brown rice

DAY 8

Breakfast

Whole wheat English muffin spread with cottage cheese and sprinkled with cinnamon

Sliced apple

1 egg, scrambled

Lunch

Turkey chili

Whole grain roll

Small side salad with 2 tablespoons oil and vinegar dressing

Dinner

Grilled or broiled wild salmon brushed with 1 teaspoon olive oil

Quinoa tossed with diced apples and sunflower seeds in 1 tablespoon walnut oil

Steamed or grilled asparagus sprinkled with Parmesan cheese

DAY 9

Breakfast

Omelet made with 1 egg plus 2 egg whites, spinach, red peppers, and organic skim mozzarella cheese, cooked in 1 teaspoon canola oil

2 slices whole wheat toast with trans-fat free margarine or butter

Lunch

Whole wheat pita pocket filled with chopped seasoned grilled chicken, roasted peppers, and mixed field greens and drizzled with 1 tablespoon olive oil and balsamic vinegar

Dinner

Filet mignon (free-range organic beef, if possible)

Wild rice

Roasted vegetables tossed with 1 tablespoon olive oil

DAY 10

Breakfast

Yogurt parfait made with 6 ounces plain nonfat yogurt, chopped fruit, sunflower seeds, chopped walnuts, cinnamon, high-fiber dry cereal, a splash of soy milk, and a sprinkle of flaxseed

Lunch

Grilled cheese sandwich made with 2 slices whole grain bread, 1 slice Swiss cheese, 1 slice light Havarti cheese, sliced tomato, and baby spinach

1 cup roasted red pepper and tomato soup (or other vegetable or vegetable bean soup)

Dinner

1 broiled chicken breast seasoned with lemon, garlic, and paprika, topped with salsa and a dollop of plain yogurt

Grilled onions, peppers, zucchini, and mushrooms

½ cup brown rice

Phase III: Maintenance

If you've come this far with the diet, you are well tuned to the benefits of eating right. Now is not the time to cast aside everything that you've learned, but you can relax into a new lifestyle. If you have the occasional calorie-filled dessert or a little too much wine, your body will soon be directing you back to your new and healthier ways. You'll be looking for a balance of foods that makes you feel great and can realistically be eaten (and enjoyed!) for the rest of your life.

Basic Action

The maintenance period allows you to reintroduce some of the foods you were required to remove during the first 3 or 4 weeks. In the simplest terms, restriction doesn't do anyone any good. Just as you learned that too much of even the most healthful foods is not good for your body, neither is restriction. You shouldn't have sugary desserts every day or rich pasta dishes or wine on a regular basis, but you also shouldn't forego special occasions and foods that are especially appealing to you. Nor should you overdo any one food group—even if it is veggies! You must always seek balance.

The No More Back Pain Diet has given you a sense of well-being, and now you want to focus on keeping that feeling. When you occasionally have a treat, don't go overboard, and be sure to listen to what your body tells you the next day. If you wake up in the morning stiff and achy after a glass of red wine, you will want to steer clear of the wine next time. Or maybe you *can* have a glass of wine with dinner as long as you don't have pasta, too. These are the things that you will figure out as you begin to reintroduce foods.

During this phase, I highly recommend that you introduce foods one day at a time and keep a food journal. Be as detailed as possible in your journaling: record amounts of foods, cooking methods, and how you felt after each meal. A food journal can speak volumes about dietary habits that you may have never realized you had. It can be very eye-opening and informational.

Duration

Forever onward! This is how you'll be eating from this day on.

Now that you've completed 3 to 4 weeks of Phases I and II, you'll have learned what your body feels like when it is working optimally. This is your baseline, the way you want each and every meal and snack to make you feel. Begin to introduce foods from the nonapproved list very carefully. You may now eat all

> ## Check Out My Website
>
> Visit my website at www.thetruthaboutbackpainbook.com to find more recipes, nutrition tips, and ideas to help you stick with your eating plan.

fruits and vegetables, but reintroduce the foods slowly. If any food makes you feel less than baseline, make a point to avoid that food. Most important, remember that you do not *need* to reintroduce any of these foods. You may choose to follow the No More Back Pain Diet carefully for the rest of your life. But, realistically, many of us need to include the occasional glass of wine or pancake (foods on the nonapproved list) in our diet to stay satisfied. That is what the maintenance period is about—finding out what your body can handle and what it does not want you to do.

PART FOUR

It's All in Your Head: The Emotions and Back Pain

CHAPTER 10

Uncovering the Root of Emotion-Based Back Pain

What happens in the mind of man is always reflected
in the disease of his body.

—René Dubos

Almost every day patients come to our offices complaining of back or neck pain that we eventually diagnose as having an emotional or stress-related cause.

The best explanation that I've heard of what it means to be stressed came from one of my patients: "People who are stressed are no longer able to live in the moment. They are too worried about what has just happened and what's coming next to be able to live in—or enjoy—the present." Life stresses—and our often negative reactions to them in the form of anger, distress, or fear—are major triggers of both acute and chronic back and neck pain. The muscle tightening that occurs during waking and sleeping can result in debilitating physiological pain of the neck, shoulders, and back. Nervous stomach, tight muscles, headaches, broken-out skin, and jaw pain are also very real physical symptoms, all of which can have an emotional base.

Since the 1970s, researchers have definitively established that such mind/body connections exist. It would seem that the torture of the mind can be more painful to the back than the torture of the body. Swedish researchers have found that women who report high stress levels are more likely to suffer from back pain than people who spend their days in jobs that involve heavy lifting.

In fact, the mind and body are so interconnected that they actually make up one undivided network. When you experience a psychological (mind) imbalance—for example, when you are chronically angry about a problem at work—you also often develop a physiological (body) imbalance or pain. This type of pain is so tightly linked to our emotional state that one can even raise the proverbial chicken-or-egg question: Which comes first, the pain or the distress about the pain?

Suffering from back pain can in itself be quite stressful. Back pain sufferers wonder if they will ever be pain-free again, if they will be able to exercise or garden or travel. Some are in such pain that they worry that they will not be able to get out of bed in the morning. Unfortunately, for many people, this line of thinking turns into a self-fulfilling prophecy as the stress of the back pain itself creates more back pain. But even if you are experiencing emotional upheaval and consequently back pain, there are positive steps you can take immediately to relax and begin to feel better.

This chapter explains how your entire biochemistry affects, and is affected by, your thought patterns and emotions.

Emotional Pain Is Very Real

Most people recognize that when something upsetting happens in their lives it is normal to feel tense or sad or irritable. However, what is less often acknowledged is that if something bad happens in your life, you may have a headache, a stomachache, a backache, or even a cold. These physical symptoms often manifest several days after the bad event, so people don't always make the connection, but there is most definitely an emotional component to our physical state of health.

When a patient is hit with back pain and the doctor can't find a structural cause, we often find that the pain is both a symptom and an expression of some distress in the person's life. Unfortunately, we often hit a raw nerve when we broach this subject. Most people don't want to believe that stress can cause a back problem. They view this revelation as an indictment on their personality, such as a weakness or a flaw. We are programmed to think we are supposed to be able to handle stress, that we should be too tough to get sick or have pain from something emotional.

If you remember that our mind/body connection is like a tightly twisted rope, then it is perfectly understandable that our emotions set off two types of reactions: psychological and physiological.

The best way to explain emotional physiology is to think about a time when you had a nightmare. When you awoke you realized that you had just had a nightmare, that there is no green monster chasing you; however, the way you felt when you woke up belied the fact that you were sleeping: You may have been perspiring, your heart may have been racing, and you may have even called out or screamed during the dream. The body does not distinguish between real and perceived danger—it simply responds to what your brain, whether asleep or awake, tells it. It is this physiological response that is the key to how emotions can affect your health.

Think about how many people get rushed to the hospital complaining of chest pains only to find out that they aren't suffering a heart attack but rather are having a panic attack. Many of the symptoms are the same, except for the heart damage. The amazing thing about a panic attack is that once the patient is assured it is not a heart attack the pain often goes away.

Emotional physiology is so powerful, it can be used to prove the guilt or innocence of a person accused of a crime. For example, consider the polygraph, or lie detector test. An examiner hooks a candidate up to a machine and asks the person a series of questions. Because people become stressed out by certain questions and respond physically (albeit silently), the lie detector is able to pick up on physiologic changes when a person is not telling the truth. These machines can register many physiologic changes (such as changes in heart rate, blood pressure, and perspiration levels) that are immediately observable.

A patient named Taylor came to see me because she had woken up with severe back pain. After an examination, I found no physical cause, so I asked
Taylor if everything was going okay in her life. Immediately after I asked
her this question, tears welled up in her eyes, and she shared a personal and
troubling experience, which I felt to be the underlying cause of her current
distress.

Not surprisingly, receiving a sympathetic response to a problem often starts the
curative process. People feel much better after talking about what is really bothering them, and I generally point out to patients that if mentioning their stress
makes them cry, then just imagine what the stress is doing to their backs. As I've
pointed out, anything that will affect you psychologically will affect you physio-
logically, and that often leads to excessive muscle tightness and back pain.

What Happens When You Are Stressed?

Prolonged muscular tension brought about by emotional stress can lead to back
pain. In Chapter 2, I quoted Hans Selye, a pioneer in stress research, who said of
the body's relation to stress: "God will forgive you but your nervous system will
not." His studies focused on the fact that the body is built to handle periods of
high stress and that our reactions replicate what our ancestors needed to do to
save themselves when hunting. For example, a hunter might be alert but relaxed,
but then suddenly he encounters some form of danger, perhaps a tiger ready to
pounce. Immediately, the body tells the stress glands (the adrenals) that it is time
for fight or flight. The body will have either unbelievable strength to fight the
predator or incredible speed and endurance to run away. After the threat is gone,
the body needs to recover from that extremely stressful episode.

We now know that very specific physical changes occur when we encounter
something stressful. When we are stressed, our bodies are programmed to prepare us to respond. As a result:

- Heart rate and blood pressure soar to increase the flow of blood to the
  brain to improve decision making.

- Blood sugar rises to furnish more fuel for energy as the result of the breakdown of glycogen, fat, and protein stores.

- The blood is shunted away from the gut (and digestion stops so as not to use up energy that is needed elsewhere) to the large muscles of the arms and legs to provide more strength in combat or greater speed in getting away from a scene of potential peril.

- Blood clotting occurs more quickly to prevent blood loss from lacerations or internal hemorrhage.

These and many other automatic responses developed to facilitate our ancestors' ability to deal with physical challenges. However, the nature of stress for modern humans is not a confrontation with a saber-toothed tiger but, instead, it's getting stuck in traffic or dealing with a family or work situation. Unfortunately, our bodies react with the same fight or flight response that not only is no longer useful but, over time, can lead to chronic fatigue, digestive upset, headaches, and back pain. The cardiovascular system, the nervous system, and the immune system may be affected.

In today's world, we suffer from a steady barrage of medium levels of stress. This constant level of tension depletes our adrenal glands, and the body's constant call for adrenalin wears us out and leaves us ill-prepared to react to the next stressor we encounter.

Stress also affects the body's ability to function in unison. Think of a time when you felt completely frazzled: your brain was fried and you just couldn't get a grip on things or slow down. The layperson's diagnosis is, "My head is going too fast for my body—I can't think." While this may sound silly, it is ultimately an accurate description of what is going on.

If you are stressed out (your head is spinning from all that is going on), many muscles in your body will only contract and not relax. If this happens for a prolonged period of time, a damaging physiologic response will occur. Cerebrospinal fluid flows throughout your spine; it works in a way that's similar to the transmission fluid in your car, making sure that everything is lubricated and flowing properly. When the cerebrospinal fluid flows too fast due to stress, it irritates the vegas nerve, which controls our abdominal organs. This irritation can cause all sorts of stress reactions, from brain freeze to an upset stomach.

The Causes of Stress Reactions

Although our bodies respond physically regardless of the type of threat, people today benefit from a better understanding of the causes of stress: internal (your response is out of proportion to the actual threat), external (you're stuck in a traffic jam and there's nothing you can do about it), temporary (a brief moment passes—like that traffic jam), and chronic (long-term job dissatisfaction or family illness). Let's look at each of these types of possible sources so that you can consider where your own stress comes from.

Internal Pressures and Emotional Conflict

Emotional conflict and the pressures we place on ourselves frequently cause enough stress to manifest as back pain. Any time we dread something or don't want to do something, we can cause a bad reaction in our bodies.

It is not surprising to learn that the greatest number of heart attacks occur on Monday mornings. People respond physically to the thought of the weekend being over and the workweek beginning.

We all have things we dread. Fortunately, they don't usually cause heart attacks. Pain from an internal cause also occurs when our conscious mind and our subconscious mind are not in harmony. If you get involved in something that goes against what you subconsciously want, a back problem can easily come about.

Ken, a healthy, active 26-year-old, who had been under my care for a few years for some mild structural back pain, was the perfect patient; he would come for checkups every month just to make sure that he stayed healthy. One day I got a distressed call from him. He could barely get out of bed due to severe back pain. Ken felt that all of the previous treatments were in vain, and he was calling to fire me. We talked on the

Anniversaries Can Be Harmful to Our Health

Whenever you think of anniversaries, you frequently think of happy anniversaries; however, our minds and bodies often take note of the sad anniversaries as well. Here are two examples.

A patient entered the office with a stiff neck. After examining her and ascertaining that there had been no trauma or accident that would cause the pain, I learned that she was nearing the 1-year anniversary of when she and her boyfriend broke up. This was particularly disheartening to her because she had thought he was the love of her life, and she had yet to meet anyone new.

Another patient came to my office completely bent over from lower back pain. Her discomfort was so severe that she had great difficulty even getting on the examination table. After taking a case history and performing an examination, we were able to determine that her lower back pain was due to stress. She mentioned that her father had died the previous summer and that summer had always been their time together. The change in the seasons triggered a negative anniversary response in this patient.

phone long enough for me to encourage him to get to the office so we could see what the problem was. As I examined him, I could see that he was truly suffering. However, I couldn't find a structural reason why. We continued to talk for a while, and I explained how stress causes muscle tightness that can cause terrible pain. Was he stressed about anything in particular? It was then that he had an "aha moment." He said he was getting married in 2 weeks and had been having second thoughts. I encouraged him to do what he had to do to resolve his feelings—and his pain.

Ultimately, Ken said his back pain was the best thing that ever happened to him. As difficult as it was for him to do, he called off his wedding and hasn't had any back pain since. And Ken is not alone in this type of response to a major life event. It is not uncommon to see an increase in acute back attacks right around the holidays.

External Events, Outside Influences, and Temporary Stress

Although our external stressors today don't involve large jungle animals, we very definitely have our own living nightmares, which may be as diverse as awaiting the results of a medical test, being trapped in a plane on the tarmac for several hours, being stuck in a seemingly endless traffic jam, or waiting to hear if we're about to get a new job. Most of the stress from these types of situations comes from feeling out of control: We can't rush the medical results, we can't get off the plane or out of the traffic jam, and we have no control over the hiring practices of a corporation.

We're also subject to the emotional environment around us. Our emotions are not isolated feelings, separate and distinct from the rest of the world. In his book *Social Intelligence*, Daniel Goleman states, "[T]he brain itself is social. One person's inner state affects and drives the other person. We actually catch each other's emotions like a cold."

In essence, *other* people's emotions can make you sick. If your spouse is unemployed and having a hard time finding a job, his or her stress has an effect on you. And what do you think happens to you when your coworker gets into a big argument with his or her spouse before coming to work? That employee's negative energy and emotions can impact your day and thus your health.

Chronic Stress

Although most stress is caused by fleeting events, such as getting cut off in traffic or missing the bus, chronic stress is a different story. Those who suffer from it report that it seems as if there were no light at the end of the tunnel.

Chronic stress can arise from any number of events: a long-term family illness, a dead-end job, or a poor relationship. Although chronic stress is upsetting, you need to recognize it for what it is and begin to work at not letting it be all-encompassing. You won't find any relief at the bottom of a bottle or at the back of the refrigerator.

You need to take positive steps toward overcoming chronic stress: Volunteer on a regular basis (there's nothing like helping another person in need to get you out of your self-pitying mood), start an exercise program (even a brisk walk around the block will release endorphins that will make you feel better immediately), or find a support group to help you get through a rough patch in your life.

How Do You Start Your Day?

Do you smack your snooze button and dread getting up? Or do you listen to the morning news, then grab a cup of coffee and rush to catch a train or jump in your car so you won't be late for work?

How you start your day sets the tone for the next 24 hours.

Instead, try this: Set your alarm clock 10 minutes earlier. In the greater scheme of things, these lost 10 minutes of sleep won't affect you too much. Use that extra few minutes to do a few stretches before dressing. Then sit down to eat a healthy breakfast. It doesn't have to be elaborate, but just taking this time rather than eating on the run will make a world of difference. (Check out the breakfast suggestions in Chapter 9.)

Copy the Athlete

Have you ever heard of a professional athlete who gets ready for his or her work-day by racing to the arena and grabbing a quick cup of coffee and a sugary muffin before going out to compete? No! Athletes prepare by eating a healthy meal, arriving at the arena early, stretching, doing some slow exercises, and getting in the mind-set to compete. We need to treat our jobs and lives the way an athlete would. Don't you think that your career, your well-being, and your family's well-being deserve that type of preparation and effort from you?

How Do You End Your Day?

At the end of the day, do you plop into bed to watch some violent television program and mentally replay all that went wrong in your day? You have to feed your head with good stuff as you end your day. If not, you won't sleep well, and you will continue your cycle of being stressed out.

If you feel the quality of your sleep isn't all that it should be, here are steps to take to ensure a more restful night, which in turn will help with back pain:

- **BOTH MATTRESS SCIENCE AND PEOPLE CHANGE.** Mattresses are getting better and better, and as we age, our needs change. If your

How Relaxation Can Affect Your Muscles

Most people fail to understand the full effect emotions can have on their muscu-lature. When you are stressed, your muscles literally become tight and stiff; con-versely, when you are relaxed, your muscles are loose and flexible.

To get a rough idea of what can happen to your body, try this exercise:

1. Stand up with plenty of room around you.

2. Raise your right arm out directly in front of you.

3. With your right arm raised in this position, twist your body all the way to the right without moving your legs.

4. Make note of the farthest thing that you can see as you look to the right.

5. Now put your arm to your side and close your eyes. Take five deep and slow breaths, holding for counts of 5 seconds on both the inhala-tion and the exhalation. (This causes your body to begin to relax.)

6. Raise your right arm up again and twist like you did before, this time with your eyes closed.

7. Now open your eyes. How far can you see to your right this time?

8. Repeat on your left-hand side.

Most people will be able to see a good bit farther the second time than they could the first. Because you have permitted your body to relax with the slow and deep breathing, you will almost certainly have increased your flexibility.

mattress is more than 8 years old or is beginning to show signs of age, buy a new one. There are more supportive models available now. (For more on buying a new mattress, see pages 75–77.)

- **ARRANGE YOUR BEDROOM FOR RELAXATION.** The ideal temperature for sleeping is 60 to 65 degrees. Block outside noise with a fan or a sound machine.

- **KEEP WORK-RELATED ITEMS OUT OF THE BEDROOM.**

- **DON'T EXERCISE OR EAT TOO CLOSE TO BEDTIME.** And limit your caffeine intake late in the day.

- **GO TO BED ABOUT THE SAME TIME EACH NIGHT, AND DO SOMETHING CALMING RIGHT BEFORE BED.** Quiet reading or a calming television program (no action-adventure or suspense at bedtime!) may help you nod off.

Ending the Circle of Negativity

Unfortunately, emotional tension creates a circle of negativity: "I have a neck ache because I'm anxious, and now I'm even more anxious because this seems to be something I'm causing myself." Generally, when patients realize that their physical symptoms in response to stressful situations are normal, they begin to feel better right away. As a result, they can more productively change the way they respond to stress.

Attitude Is Key

Stanford University conducted an exhaustive and far-reaching study on the predictors of back pain by researching the workers at the Boeing Corporation. One aspect of the study involved more than 3,000 employees over many years. The study relied on physical examinations, MRI results, X-rays, and anything else that researchers thought might indicate future back pain. The study reached an important conclusion: Emotional outlook and psychological factors are the number one predictor of back pain!

Chapter 11 offers advice on daily living habits that can make a big difference in attitude and back pain.

Attitudes and Exercises That Heal

Stress doesn't change. Combined, my father and I have seen countless patients for almost 60 years, and my father could have attested to the fact that times change but emotional tension doesn't. In the 1970s, people came to my father's practice for relief from neck pain, tight shoulders, upper back tension, lower back pain, and back spasms, just as they come to the practice today.

So if stress doesn't change, what can we alter to make the situation better?

You can change how your body responds to it. To help you avoid getting tight through the shoulders, the neck, or the lower back and discovering that you can't get out of bed one morning because the pain is so severe, this chapter provides ways to deflect the emotional pressure you feel. Feeling good and being pain-free involves learning to unwind before going to bed so that you can sleep through the night. Then, instead of sleepless nights because of pain or the need to pop painkillers to get through the day at work, you'll learn to relax and take things as they come.

Stress and the Back

People cope with anxiety differently. Everyone becomes stressed by different factors, and we each physically manifest tension in our own way—from headaches and back pain to stomach pain and upset. If 85 percent of Americans suffer back pain at some point in their lives, then it is very clear that a good number of people tighten up through their backs when they are stressed!

I often tell patients that just like building physical strength, building emotional strength takes training. "Train like Rocky Balboa!" we tell our patients when we are encouraging them to get into emotional shape to better handle their stress. Through attitude adjustment, better life-management skills, and some helpful ways to relax, you can learn to deal with stress. You can't always control what happens to you, but you can learn to control how you handle it, which will have a direct effect on your emotions.

A Possibly Good Thing About Back Pain

Stress and tension have to go somewhere. If your stress is manifested as tension in the muscles, then that is often preferable to having it become an internal problem that can lead to severe stomach problems or even a deadly heart attack. People who keep their emotions all bottled up often suffer unseen health issues; if you have back pain, at least you know the stress exists.

"Life is 10 percent what happens to you and 90 percent how you react to it" was a favorite saying of former football coach Lou Holtz, who guided four different teams to top 20 rankings. Change is a part of living, and it is up to us to adapt to circumstances that cannot be altered. This definitely helps keep minor annoyances at bay, but it also helps with some of life's more difficult challenges. If you consider a stressful situation in a broader context—job loss can lead to new opportunity; illness can create new family bonds—you'll find that the upsetting developments will be easier to take in stride.

The 15 Laws for Your Best Life

There are just as many ways to help you reduce the stress in your life as there are causes. Although learning to respond to stressful situations appropriately may be the key, knowing how to create an environment for yourself in which injury and pain are least likely to take hold is of paramount importance.

Law 1: Take care of yourself.

If you don't take care of yourself, you won't be able to take care of anyone else. For your health and well-being, place a priority on taking care of number one: you.

It's vital that you pay attention to your health and well-being. Eat right (see Part III), and build in time for exercise each day. In addition, set aside time to do something pleasant; we all deserve time to read or watch a favorite television show or just sit down with our kids. Think of the things you love and make a list. Over time, you ought to make time for each one.

Law 2: Match your actions to your needs.

Time is our most precious asset. Although work, family, and sleep take up much of our day, you can usually squeeze in time for yourself if you set your mind to it.

In the movie *City Slickers*, Curly (played by Jack Palance) says, "Life is about one thing, and that one thing is for you to figure out." He reminds us that we all have to choose what is most important to us and then make that our personal priority.

Part of this will involve learning to say no. If you don't want to take on a volunteer project after work or you don't want to spend yet another weekend helping out at the in-laws, find ways to decline.

You need to bring your life into congruence. Your actions need to match what you really want. Otherwise you feel guilty—and guilt leads to stress, and stress leads to pain. If you really want to lose weight, stop eating that hot fudge sundae because this incongruence (what you want = weight loss vs. what you do = consume a high-calorie dessert) is going to give you back pain. If you really hate your job, start looking for a new one. Otherwise, back and neck pain will continue. The pain you feel is the consequence of not dealing with what is really going on. Stop the self-sabotage; develop a plan that will make you happy.

Law 3: Build positive personal connections.

Friends help us live longer. If you are single and live far from family, a strong friendship—or group of friends—can work wonders for your health. Accepting help and support from those who care about you and listen helps you develop that all-important positive outlook.

Study after study has revealed that social ties reduce our risk of disease by lowering blood pressure, heart rate, and cholesterol levels. A recent University of California at Los Angeles (UCLA) study on friendship among women documented the importance of such female-to-female relationships, and scientists are now beginning to explore ways to prove that women's response to stress often includes brain chemicals that encourage the creation of social links for support in times of need.

Dr. Laura Cousin Klein, one of the study's lead authors, notes that it may be part of an ancient survival mechanism: When the hormone oxytocin is released, which often happens at times of stress, it encourages the gathering of friends and family as part of a calming response.

Law 4: Slow down.

Frequently a patient will speed-walk into my office, as if walking more quickly would let him or her get more done. Slow down. Chill out. Remember the song that goes, "Slow down, you move too fast / You got to make the mornin' last"? My patients just love it when I sing this to them. (Their smiles don't tell me whether they are laughing at me or with me, but in any case, at least they are smiling!)

I frequently prescribe this for patients: "Walk more slowly; drive more slowly; notice the passing scenery; take deep breaths. I guarantee you'll feel better."

Law 5: Don't minimize the positives or maximize the negatives.

Feeling positive decreases stress, and positive feelings have to start from within. I often observe that women, particularly, are dismissive of their opportunities to shine. For example, if someone compliments a woman on a dress she's wearing, she is likely to respond with a comment along the lines of "This old thing?" or "I couldn't find anything else this morning," or an unenthusiastic, "Oh, thanks." Men tend to grunt and are also likely to barely hear a compliment.

Next time, instead of blowing off such a nice moment, let it be your opportunity to radiate positive feelings! Take in a compliment like inhaling a breath of fresh air. Then exhale the positive feelings that come when someone says, "You look nice!"

In general, it's vital to nurture a positive view of yourself. Acknowledging your own strength and resourcefulness in dealing with difficult times can help you develop confidence in yourself.

Although many people are poor at accepting compliments, most of us tend to blow out of proportion any kind of negative remark. When an employee goes through an annual review with the human resources department and is given overall positive feedback and a couple of things to work on, I often find that employee on my chiropractic table with back pain. He or she is worrying and worrying over the couple of things that could use improvement but is not thinking about the positive aspects of the performance review. Learn to take negative feedback in stride. If you consider it and find it valid, then think about how to change. If you consider it and find it without merit, then toughen up. None of us is going to be beloved by everyone we come across.

Law 6: Let go.

We all worry—it's human nature—but we could all spend less time at it! The word *worry* originates from a Middle English word that originally meant "to strangle" or "to choke." If you think about it, worrying is actually a way we strangle ourselves. We cut off our air passages to feeling better, acting naturally, and relaxing.

The best way to stop worrying is simply to recognize that you are worried about something and let yourself have 3 to 5 minutes to consider what you are worried about: For example, you have a new boss, and this makes you nervous. Once you acknowledge this concern, don't worry—just focus on doing a great job. You'll work better if you eliminate your concerns, and chances are that everything will be fine once the adjustment is made. Or perhaps your child is walking to school with a group of peers for the first time. Well, if you've already walked the route with him, you've talked with him about street safety, and you know and like the group he's walking with, you just have to let go. Most of the things that we stress about don't come to pass, and most of the time we don't have any control over what we are worrying about anyway!

Absolutely do not worry about what you can't control. If you have no control over a situation, then turn in your "in-charge card." I used to be a nervous flier until someone pointed out that there was no sense in worrying because there was nothing I could do to make it safer. If I make the decision to get on the plane, I have no control over what happens next, so I might as well lean back in my seat and enjoy the down time. Make this your mantra: "If I can't control it, I won't sweat it." You'll be surprised at the number of situations that will improve once you realize this.

Law 7: Take a break.

Seriously! Even a long weekend will give you some badly needed R and R. You would be amazed by how much better your back can feel if you just recharge your batteries. Take time out or go on vacation. A change of scenery for even a few days can make a big difference.

And in the evening, disconnect from stress—turn off your BlackBerry, cell phone, and laptop. People are feeling more and more that they can't do that, but you should try to once in a while. If your job is so critical that you have to stay connected, put a firm limit on the time you spend at home responding to emails and phone calls.

Law 8: Recognize and acknowledge the problem.

Admitting you have a problem is always the first step to healing. If you think it's a sign of weakness to admit you have a problem—whether it's difficulty at home or troubles at work, it's important to remember that everyone has problems!

The test of strength or weakness has to do with how you handle problems—do you struggle to find a solution or do you let the problem get the better of you?

Law 9: Take decisive action.

Consider what is happening to make you stressed and how you might approach the problem. Instead of wishing an issue or a problem would go away, take steps toward a solution. The early steps are generally small steps, but slowly you will begin to increase your stride toward a solution.

If something in your life has proven to be disruptive (illness or job change), establish new routines as soon as you can, and you'll begin to feel better.

Law 10: Avoid seeing crises as insurmountable problems.

You can't undo certain pieces of misfortune (death of a relative, illness, damage from a storm), but you can change how you react to them. Try to see beyond the current crisis. Note any subtle ways in which you might already feel somewhat better as you deal with difficult situations.

Law 11: Take time to reflect.

Pausing to reflect on what is happening can give you a better perspective on it. Whether the solution for you is meditation, praying, or long solitary walks, find a way to think through what is bothering you. Meditation and spiritual practices help some people build connections and restore hope. Others write in their journals about their deepest thoughts relating to the trauma or other stressful event.

Law 12: Read a self-help book.

Read books to help you cope. I frequently recommend the book *Anatomy of an Illness as Perceived by the Patient*, by Norman Cousins, but there are many other helpful books. A few others I've enjoyed are *Goals!*, by Brian Tracy; *A Better Way to Live*, by Og Mandino; *Fresh Start Promise*, by my good friend Edwige Gilbert; and *Awaken the Giant Within*, by Anthony Robbins. There are also self-help books written to help get people through a specific type of difficulty, from surviving divorce to overcoming financial ruin to parenting a difficult child.

A good book will offer practical advice and reasons to be motivated—and will be the kind of reference you can return to again and again.

Law 13: Fall in Love

When you are in love, nothing hurts! And if you've already got someone, then "love the one you're with!" And have sex. Humans need touch and intimate interactions. I love the *Seinfeld* moment when George describes parking as being like sex: If you really apply yourself, you can get it for free.

Law 14: Keep a sense of humor.

Humor is so important in this world. Watch a comedy on television, read something funny, or take a lesson from my wife and sleep with someone funny-looking. It's guaranteed to keep you smiling.

Law 15: Consult a mental health professional.

There is nothing wrong with seeking professional help. According to a report in the January 2007 issue of *Health Psychology*, psychological help, when offered alone or as part of multidisciplinary treatment, had a definite effect on pain intensity and quality of life. The most effective types of therapy for back pain were cognitive behavioral therapy and self-regulatory therapy (biofeedback and relaxation).

If you suffer chronic back pain, you may also be suffering from depression. One fascinating study found that taking a low dose of a tricyclic antidepressant soothed nerves in the back enough to cut pain in up to 60 percent of patients.

Although I generally favor a non-medication approach to becoming pain-free, I have observed that patients who start taking an antidepressant prescribed by a mental health professional slowly decrease their need for other types of pain-relief medications.

Judi had been coming to us monthly for several years with chronic lower back pain and overall stiffness. Regardless of the treatments we provided, Judi never felt 100 percent, and she became resigned to the fact that it was just her nature to be tight and stiff due to her age and sedentary lifestyle. One day when she came into the office for her monthly adjustment, she reported that she was completely pain-free. I asked her what caused such a remarkable improvement. She said that she had been suffering from some mild depression, and her primary care doctor put her on a low-level antidepressant. This antidepressant had changed her life by finally banishing the tension she habitually carried in her back.

Because a primary cause of back pain is emotional, it makes good sense that an antidepressant can have a profound impact on back pain—providing that the person's back pain stems from an emotional cause in the way that Judi's did.

Although I believe a drug-free approach should always be the first choice, some emotional issues are overpowering, and we encourage you to stick with the medications that your mental healthcare provider has recommended. Plus, I would rather have you on an antidepressant than popping anti-inflammatory medication or muscle relaxants on a regular basis

Build Resilience

Resilience is the process of adapting well in the face of adversity, trauma, tragedy, threats, or other significant sources of stress (such as family and relationship problems, serious health problems, and workplace and financial troubles). It means bouncing back from difficult experiences. We all need this inner strength. The very nature of human existence means that we are going to encounter difficulties at least some of the time.

In our practice, we've noted that the number of times that someone has been knocked down by family difficulties or job loss, for example, is less important than the manner in which he or she keeps getting up. We see some patients who have been fired because of the sale of their company, have lost spouses, and have helped elderly parents through long illnesses, but they still have very sunny outlooks on the future. It's not just about being Pollyanna. It's about being able to face challenges, changing what you can, and moving on. Your public library is filled with thousands of stories of successful people overcoming defeats and setbacks and going on to reach unparalleled heights of success. Staying down is not a very inviting possibility, so you might as well fight to be among those who bounce back.

Here are four ways to build resilience:

1. Maintain a hopeful outlook.
Try to visualize what you want rather than worrying about what you fear. An optimistic outlook enables you to expect that good things will happen in your life.

Studies on everything from heart disease to cancer show that a positive outlook can make a big difference in survival rate. And, of course, remember that the Stanford and Boeing study cited earlier noted that the number one predictor of future back pain was emotional outlook. When we are happy, our bodies exude different chemicals than when we are worried or sad. So let those wonderful endorphins flow through your body, and you'll benefit in the long run. With further study, scientists will likely learn that these hormones trigger some level of healing.

2. Set goals and keep your eye on the prize.

Develop some realistic goals, and then outline small steps you can take to achieve them. Each week, take at least one small step toward your long-term goal. For example, if you want to go back to school for an advanced degree, an early and small step would simply be finding out about the requirements: What preparatory courses or what testing is needed to qualify? A phone call or an Internet search, either of which could be accomplished in under 30 minutes, would provide you with a list of additional small steps to take on the way to the larger goal. Even if it seems like a small accomplishment, you'll begin to realize that small steps are leading you forward. Instead of focusing on the ultimate goal, once a week ask yourself, "What's one thing I know I can accomplish today that helps me move in the direction I want to go?"

3. Look for opportunities for self-discovery.

Adversity sometimes has its benefits—not that you wouldn't prefer to avoid it, but people often learn something about themselves and others and may find that they have grown in some respect as a result of difficulty or stress. For example, I know one family whose daughter had to have kidney surgery, and they found an outpouring of kindness from the community as well as incredibly caring and devoted medical professionals. While they would prefer to have not had to go through what they did, the kindness and respect they received throughout was heartening. The girl is now a very kind and caring teenager, and one can't help but think that this experience had something to do with it.

When people who have experienced tragedies and hardship are later interviewed, they report a heightened appreciation for life with a renewed sense of self-worth, a more developed spirituality, better relationships, and a greater sense of strength as a result of what they lived through. Because you don't usually have a say in bad luck happening, you might as well look for that sort of silver lining. There almost always is one.

Stress Levels

The magazine *Men's Health* recently published a stress scale that analyzed the following stressors and their attendant increase in stress levels:

- An overbearing boss will increase your stress levels by 110 percent.

- Drinking coffee will increase your stress levels by 32 percent.

- A tight deadline will increase your stress levels by 45 percent.

- A driving commute will increase your stress levels by 80 percent.

- Late nights at the office will increase your stress levels by 270 percent.

Conversely, the article noted that in addition to mind/body relaxation exercises, the following can lead to a reduction in overall stress levels:

- A happy marriage will reduce your stress levels by 55 percent.

- Listening to soothing music 25 minutes per day will reduce your stress levels by 25 percent.

- Exercising on a treadmill 30 minutes per day will reduce your stress levels by 17 percent.

- Meditating will reduce your stress levels by 44 percent.

- Having sex will reduce your stress levels by 15 percent.

- Watching a comedy will reduce your stress levels by 98 percent.

4. Give back.

No matter how bad your stress, the chances are excellent that someone else is in a lot worse shape than you are. If you've got a roof over your head, food on the table, and someone to call when you are down, then you have much to be grateful for. (A single visit to a pediatric oncology ward should be enough to rid you of any woe-is-me feelings.) I have heard from countless friends, family members, and patients that what I have learned for myself is true for them as well. If you can find a few minutes each week or each month to volunteer to help someone out, you'll begin to feel better. Our office does a lot of work for the Make-A-Wish Foundation; when I help out, I find that all of my problems suddenly seem very small. If you have no particular place where you would like to volunteer, conduct an Internet search through sites such as www.volunteermatch.org. I read of one organization that needs people to occasionally call homebound senior citizens. All you need is a few spare minutes and your cell phone for that—and you *will* feel better.

Some Relaxation Exercises

All people, whether a highly compensated CEO or a stay-at-home mom, are sub-ject to stress. Some of those people may have the time or resources to indulge in long vacations, leisurely walks in the park, or 90-minute yoga classes. For the rest of us, the following brief exercises will help get you through the next hour, the day, the next week . . .

The Thinker

Find a quiet spot (close your office door). Sit comfortably and close your eyes. (If you wear glasses, take them off for this exercise.) Press the fingertips of both hands lightly along the ridge above your brow. Take four or five slow breaths.

For something that takes less than a minute to do, this little exercise provides a surprising amount of relaxation—bringing with it a sense of calm. The genesis of this exercise actually comes from something we all do anyway. When we are upset or troubled, we tend to rub our forehead, an instinctual reaction that is physically beneficial. In Asian medicine, it is believed that the forehead is the emotional center.

Deep Breathing

Here's an easy one: deep breathing. What could be easier than that? (It's actually not as easy as you think if you are stressed!) The yogis know what they are doing when they place a big emphasis on "breath with motion." Just simply taking full deep breaths, inhaling and exhaling completely, is extremely cleansing and calm-ing. When people become stressed, their breathing rate speeds up; to relax, they need to slow that rate down. Fortunately, it's quite easy to accomplish.

There are many breathing techniques that can act as stress reducers. Although there are entire books written on proper breathing (and lots of parodies of breathing in movies and on TV), the breathing technique that we have found the most useful is also quite simple.

- Inhale slowly for a count of 4.
- Hold it for a count of 4.
- Exhale for a count of 4.

At first, do this exercise for just 2 minutes. As you breathe, empty your mind of all thoughts—or if thoughts creep in, let them pass. Over time, try to extend the amount of time you devote to this relaxing practice.

Relaxation Pose

One of the most relaxing positions in yoga, and a method that can be curative for migraines, involves lying on your back with your legs extended up the wall. Sitting with one hip aligned as close to the wall as possible, swing your legs up as you lie back so that both legs are extended up the wall and there is no space between your buttocks and the wall. Lie in this position for 10 minutes or so. Not only does this inversion increase blood flow to the torso, but it also allows the muscles along your spine to fully relax.

Walking

A study of back patients revealed that walking was not only a great stress reliever but also helpful in relieving back pain. Half the patients were given exercises intended to strengthen the lower back; the other half were told to get out and walk regularly. Just 30 days later, the walkers reported less stress and more pain relief.

You don't have to power walk, but you should wear sensible footwear and make the process as comfortable and invigorating as possible. Walk alone and introduce a contemplative aspect to your outing, or walk with a partner, your child in a stroller, or your dog to keep you company.

Listen to the Tahitian Fisherman

When my wife and I were honeymooning in Bora Bora, we took a boat trip with a big group of people who were all going snorkeling. I was speaking to the boat operator, and I asked if he liked what he did. He looked at me as if it were the stupidest question he had ever heard, and his response was something I will never forget: "If I didn't like it, why would I do it?"

I explained that where I came from, most people don't like what they do. He answered bluntly, "That's stupid."

If your job is giving you a pain in the back, it's probably not just ergonomics. Because so much stress is job-related, doesn't it make sense that if you don't like your job, you should do something about it? Either change your attitude or change your job. But change for change's sake won't remove the stress. It's the way you deal with the stress of the job that matters.

You decide which techniques will work best for you to reduce stress and the back pain it can cause. But making these stress-free exercises part of your daily routine will generate incomparable results.

CHAPTER 12

Circulating Energy: A New Look at Chinese Medicine

One of the problems with Western medicine is that it is becoming less and less personal. Patients are treated like defective robots, and we are supposed to go to the right specialist to get the problem taken care of. If you have a heart problem, you see a heart specialist; and once that problem is fixed, that doctor is pretty much done with you. You may still have other health problems, but as far as the cardiologist is concerned, it's on to the next patient.

Chapters 10 and 11 focused on Western medical philosophy and back pain remedies in relation to stress, but given the popularity of some alternative and Eastern medical beliefs, I would be remiss if I didn't address them. Chinese medicine may hold a cure for you.

Asian medicine is offered by some professionals who hold traditional medical degrees as well as by those who are trained practitioners in Eastern techniques. The Americanized version of Asian medicine is generally both gentle and personal. Perhaps because it is often offered by those who are practicing alternative medicine, the emphasis tends to be very patient-centered, and that alone may be healing.

Though today's scientists have difficulty explaining *how* Chinese medicine works, current studies verify that it *does* work—and works quite well. I have seen some of my own patients benefit greatly from acupressure, acupuncture, and the practice of tai chi, so let me tell you a little about the Eastern philosophy of pain.

It's About the Chi

Like any type of good medical philosophy, Chinese medicine is not one-dimensional. Though we hear mostly about acupuncture, Chinese practitioners have a broad belief in considering the overall lifestyle of the patient. Depending on the issue about which the patient has consulted them, they consider a patient's diet and exercise regimen. Acupuncture, acupressure, certain types of massage, and some types of herbal healing may be recommended.

Chinese medical philosophy is rooted in the belief that the body has a motivating energy that moves through a series of channels called meridians. This energy flow is called *chi*, which is defined as "life force." In India, there is a similar belief that focuses on chakras. For thousands of years, Eastern cultures have studied, spoken about, and used this energy form. Tai chi masters—people who have mastered control of their chi—show amazing demonstrations of strength. A master might barely touch another person, and yet that person could feel as if he or she had been hit with a baseball bat.

If we are feeling well, the energy flow is like a quickly flowing river with few detours. However, when we become stressed, this flow of energy through our bodies gets blocked, throwing off our energy balance, or chi. This imbalance can lead to anything from general irritability to serious pain.

If we go back to the explanation of what happens to our bodies under stress, you'll recall that our muscles are supposed to contract and relax continuously. However, they quit relaxing when we are stressed out. As a result of stress, the muscles go into long-term contraction, which our bodies feel as neck or back tension, spasm, and pain. Chinese medicine sees the cure as getting the chi flowing again. Eastern doctors use acupressure and acupuncture to unblock the chi, and they recommend diet and exercise (such as tai chi) to maintain balance once it is righted again.

Contemporary scientific studies have shown that our bodies use many different sorts of energy. The power needed to toss a basketball is different from the energy requirements of digesting a bowl of cereal. The brain creates small amounts of electricity to pass down to the nerves and stimulate the muscles, and this electricity is created by a large number of small cellular "micro-batteries" inside the skull. But this is a new view of how our bodies work. To traditional Eastern practitioners, bodily action is explained as a continuous life force flowing through the body and keeping us alive. Keeping the chi flowing was and still is the goal of life and the measure of good health.

Though studies have proven that Chinese treatments can be very effective, scientists have yet to fully understand the reasons why. One school of thought focuses on the impact electromagnetic energy has on the body. The presence of electromagnetic energy within our bodies is well documented, and it is the basis of MRI. Norwegian scientist Dr. Bjorn Nordenstrom studied electromagnetic energy and found that the traditional Chinese meridians are apparently electromagnetic. This seems to correlate with what the Chinese have described as our overall system of energy.

The Chi in Balance

Your daily experiences, both negative and positive, affect your chi. When you listen to the morning news about terror threats, murders, household fires, and other tragedies, your chi is negatively affected. When you listen to classical music and do deep-breathing exercises or take a brisk walk, your chi is positively affected. Remember, too, that how we react to different experiences depends on what is going on in our life at that moment. The example that I always use is eating ice cream. If you are eating a hot fudge sundae to celebrate an accomplishment, it can positively affect your chi. However, eating a hot fudge sundae when you are bored and depressed about your weight will have the opposite effect.

As you might guess, relaxed musculature lets the chi flow properly. If our bodies are stress-free, then our energy is flowing and we have no need for an external means to unblock anything. If you are generally relaxed, then a day at the beach, deep breathing, a massage, a trip to the movies, a break with a hot fudge sundae, or regular exercise may be enough to keep your chi flowing freely. Once in a while, I see a patient who needs a "prescription" for a ski vacation. The fellow had terrible lower back pain, and after I provided a full examination and considered all of his issues, I surmised that his pain stemmed from some difficult political issues at his office. I told him, "Get out of here. Go skiing. Take it slow at first, and you'll be fine." And he was. Getting away from the work stress and doing what he loved was curative.

The crux of this lesson is that you need to improve the aspects of your life that will have a positive effect on your chi, and you need to decrease the experiences that will adversely affect your inner energy. These solutions are unique to you.

Acupressure and Acupuncture: Correcting Imbalance

In traditional Chinese medicine, there is no distinction between the mind and the body. The Chinese believe that restorative methods such as acupressure and acupuncture are curative for both somatic (of the body) and psychological disorders. In China, acupuncture is sometimes used instead of anesthesia.

There are a variety of points on the human body at which the underlying flow of chi can be blocked—a good number of which have a direct correlation to points on the spine. These points were mapped out thousands of years ago and have been used in acupuncture treatment ever since. The exact number of points varies from school to school and from historic period to historic period, but most practitioners today act on at least 600 points, spaced relatively evenly over the surface of the body. Stimulation may be by hand (massotherapy or acupressure) or needles (acupuncture) or heat (referred to as *moxibustion*, after the species name of the wormwood plant, an herb that is normally burned to provide the heat).

Acupressure

Have you ever had a massage that completely relaxed you? During a good massage, you are awake but still feel some sleep-like relaxing qualities. As you get up, you realize that you are at a completely different state of relaxation. What happened during this massage is that you completely changed your chi.

A massage or a specialized acupressure treatment by a trained practitioner can be extraordinarily healing. James Durlacher wrote a wonderful book called *Freedom from Fear Forever*, in which he describes a self-help method of acupressure. Such forms of acupressure can help reduce stress. Here's a really easy, do-at-the-office acupressure exercise that I love.

Golf Ball Acupressure

For this easy exercise, you need one golf ball.

Sit down in a comfortable chair and take off your shoes. Place the golf ball on the floor and rest your foot on top of the ball. Roll the ball under your foot from heel to arch to toes in a circular motion for a couple of minutes. Repeat on the other foot.

The exercise massages your foot, putting pressure on acupressure points. Your entire body will relax as you work your foot. This is a form of reflexology.

Acupuncture

Acupuncture involves the insertion of fine needles along the meridians (energy channels) to reestablish the energy flow (creating *de qi*, a dull ache, tingling, or numbness), restore balance, and encourage healing. It became popular in the West in the 1970s, after President Richard Nixon received treatment during his news-making visit to China.

The needles are left in place for approximately 40 minutes, and they may be manipulated by hand by the practitioner or stimulated with electricity. Although this sounds like a bit of an ordeal, it's actually quite relaxing. Patients may be treated as often as a couple of times a week at first and then less frequently as the pain improves. The cost ranges from $50 to $150 a session and is covered by some insurers.

It used to be thought that energy flows only in the traditionally identified channels, but over time, practitioners have found that they can affect the body positively by pinpointing an ever-expanding number of acupuncture points. Modern science reveals that a web of connective tissue supports our body's organs and other tissues. As a result, there seems to be a broader array of options of where the needles can be inserted. These points are usually where connective tissues bundle together, often around the joints. When an acupuncture needle is

A Glossary of Acupuncture Terms

- **ACUPRESSURE.** Pressure and massage are used at key points on the body to rebalance or unblock the flow of energy.

- **ACUPUNCTURE.** Traditional method of Chinese medicine in which fine needles are inserted into the body at key points to rebalance or unblock the flow of energy.

- **AURICULAR.** Pertaining to the ear.

- **CHI OR QI.** Chinese word for the life force or vital energy of the universe (pronounced *CHEE*).

- **CUPPING.** A technique that draws chi and blood to the surface of the skin via a vacuum created inside a glass cup.

- **MERIDIAN.** Channel through which vital energy flows in the body.

- **POINTS.** Access points to a person's energy system; specific places where energy flowing through the meridians can be adjusted.

inserted into the tissue, endorphins are released. A small inflammatory response is triggered, and as a result, physiological changes occur. It is speculated that the process of the small sting of the needle may prohibit passage of stronger pain signals and that that is one of the reasons why acupuncture is successful.

Although rare, there are slight risks in acupuncture, such as bruising or infection. For that reason, it's very important to get a referral from a doctor or to locate a licensed practitioner. Licensing requirements vary by state, but one major licensing body is the nonprofit National Certification Commission for Acupuncture and Oriental Medicine (www.nccaom.org). To find a medical doctor trained in acupuncture, check out the American Academy of Medical Acupuncture (www.medicalacupuncture.org).

Acupuncture for pain relief has been subjected to rigorous study in recent years. One study funded by the National Institutes of Health (NIH) concerned knee pain from osteoarthritis. It is interesting that the results proved that both real acupuncture and placebo acupuncture were helpful; the real acupuncture showed a modest edge in improving pain. One explanation for the success of the placebo procedure is that there is no real way to fake acupuncture because concerned practitioners inserted fine needles into the skin of both groups of study subjects. Until a better testing method is created, the take-away point is that the NIH studies prove that acupuncture is effective in combating pain.

Tai Chi

Tai chi chuan originated in China as one of the martial arts. It involves dozens of postures and gestures performed in sequences known as sets. Tai chi cleanses the body's tissue of accumulated stress and, by so doing, boosts all aspects of our health systems. Today it serves as a healthful, low-impact, noncompetitive series of flowing movements that move the body slowly through positions of energy balance.

Documented benefits of tai chi include boosting the immune system's strength and reducing the incidence of depression, anxiety, and chronic pain. Tai chi masters are quite skilled and have learned to harness their energy in such a way that they can perform superhuman feats. The most common example of this harnessed energy is when an experienced practitioner in one of the more combative martial arts breaks through multiple two-by-fours or concrete blocks with a single blow and without self-injury. These types of demonstrations are always remarkable, especially for someone who is completely unfamiliar with chi. But you don't need to be a tai chi master to learn to use your chi to improve your health.

Because tai chi is low impact and low stress, it can be done by anyone, almost anywhere, and no special clothing or equipment is needed. Although it takes years to build expertise in the slow flow of the series of movements, beginners can benefit immediately. Studies have shown an increase in mental relaxation and a drop in blood pressure by those who commit to this form of exercise. Studies at the Oregon Research Institute in Eugene and the Hong Kong Polytechnic University have found that tai chi can improve the sense of balance in older people and drastically reduce the risk of falls. Practiced over a period of time, an individual becomes more relaxed, gains better balance, gains greater concentration, and increases conscious circulation of vital energy through the body. Since tai chi chuan and other Chinese exercises involve systematic mental programs of mood and mood training, it is only natural that they should produce this relaxation response among practitioners.

Tai chi is popular enough that chances are you can find an instructor in your community. During good weather, many groups practice in parks or other outdoor venues. To find a teacher, check the website of the International Taoist Tai Chi Society (www.taoist.org). Or consult the American Tai Chi Association (www.americantaichi.net) for how you can incorporate simple but meaningful practices into your daily life.

Try tai chi for yourself with these simple introductory exercises:

Hugging the Tree

This is a good way to help your life force energy (chi) flow more freely throughout your body.

Stand in an alert but relaxed position, with your knees slightly bent, feet shoulder-width apart, hands at your sides. Breathe in and out slowly for 10 repetitions, allowing your mind to become clear and calm. Now raise your arms as if you were hugging a big round tree. Hold your arms in this position and continue to breathe normally for about 30 seconds while visualizing the flow of energy between your hands. Shake out your arms and repeat 3 more times.

Awaken the Chi

This exercise is a great way to stimulate your energy and, at the same time, slow you down and allow you to get centered by increasing your flexibility and correcting your breathing pattern.

Stand with your feet shoulder-width apart and parallel, toes pointing straight out. With your body erect but not stiff (imagine your head is being held up by a string from the crown), tuck your chin in slightly, relax your shoulders, and keep your gaze forward and steady.

Let your arms hang loosely at your sides, fingers curved naturally with the palms facing your body. Tuck in your tailbone and stand with your knees relaxed. Breath out as you let your body sink down, allowing your knees to bend slightly. Breathe in as you rise up and draw your arms up to shoulder height, palms facing down, elbows and wrists slightly bent. Turn your hands so the palms face out to the front, keeping your fingers curved naturally.

Breathe out as you allow your body to sink down again, bending your knees slightly. Draw your arms down to your sides with the palms facing to the back. Breathe in and raise your body up and stand with your palms facing your thighs. Repeat this sequence three times.

Bringing About Balance

The key to gaining balanced energy is figuring out how to affect and control your chi on a daily basis. Review the information in Part IV, and think about what steps you can take in your day-to-day life that will affect your chi positively. Consider how you start your morning. Every day you have a choice as to how to live your life—make the choice for less stress, less pain, and balanced chi.

If balancing your chi does not feel like enough for you, don't hesitate to seek professional help. Often short-term therapy can be very beneficial, and what is most important is to deal with your emotions to the best of your ability.

The Natural Laws
of Back Health

The more you know, the more you find out how little
you know.
—DR. SHELDON SINETT

In our practice, each day starts with a new pursuit of the why of back pain, and we work hard to find new ways to help people become pain-free. From the first day of his 46-year practice until the day he died, my dad continually worked to learn how to help more people. He never pretended to have all of the answers, but his thirst for knowledge is what led to this book.

I hope you'll continue to refer to the book for help on an as-needed basis. But as you conclude your first reading, I want to remind you of the basic messages I've discussed throughout.

Listen to Your Body

When your back or neck starts bothering you, embrace the pain and listen to what your body is telling you. Over time—and through a process of elimination—you will almost certainly reach an "aha moment" concerning your pain.

Remember the Three Causes of Back Pain

Throughout the book you've been introduced to the three main factors that can be the cause of back pain: structural, chemical, and emotional. This can all be summed up with the three natural laws of back health:

1. **BE ACTIVE AND WORK TO KEEP FLEXIBLE.** A sedentary lifestyle will leave you susceptible to injury and illness.

2. **EAT HEALTHY FOODS.** Good, wholesome food, eaten in moderation, eliminates inflammation, aids digestion, and is the key to feeling well.

3. **LEARN TO HANDLE STRESS.** Every day dedicate yourself to finding ways to relax—to relieve the tension that leads to tight muscles and back pain.

The cause of back pain is almost always multifaceted. If you address only one aspect of the three possible factors—structural, chemical, or emotional—you may not get to the root of your problem.

The triad of back health is dynamic, and each aspect is constantly in flux. If one side is compromised, the other sides will be affected as well. One reason our remedies can be effective is that they address more than one cause at a time. Consider the simple 30-minute walk: Studies show that walking does more to decrease back pain than almost any other cure. The explanation is clear: A 30-minute walk provides a full-body workout; it can also improve circulation and relieve stress. And when you introduce a healthy diet to this easy exercise regimen, you have the added benefit of good digestion, which means you are working from the outside in *and* the inside out to achieve perfect balance and total back pain relief.

We are certain that our three natural laws of back health will change the way the world views back pain. Let this book be your guide as you begin your journey to better health.

Acknowledgments

My heartfelt and enduring thanks to:

A wonderful writer, Kate Kelly, who made all this possible.

An amazing agent, Cathy Hemming.

Toni Markiet, for your help and input.

Rachel Kahan, for believing in us. You are a wonderful person and friend. All the success that comes from this book is because of you.

John Duff, Jeanette Shaw, and the entire team at Perigee, for taking a chance on a first-time author.

Dr. George Goodheart, who not only cured my dad from back pain and changed my family's life, but also changed our fundamental approach to health-care forever. The practice that my father started and that I am privileged to continue was inspired by your teachings, as was this book. We offer you our gratitude, and that of many thousands of patients who have benefited from your genius.

Dr. Peter Ottone, for reviewing the manuscript of this book and contributing his expertise—and for his lifelong friendship.

Dr. Rob Shire and Dr. Erin Cranstoun, for their support and help.

Dr. Crystal Joseph and Rachel Williams, physical therapist.

Our patients, for without you we are nothing. The journey to health has been enlightened by each and every one of you.

The partners of CJ Nutrition, for their help with the diet and for contributing many other nuggets of invaluable information.

My second family, the staff at Midtown Chiropractic Health and Wellness, with whom it is a joy and pleasure to work.

My loving wife, for allowing me to take on this endeavor and for putting up with me for the last 10 years.

My most wonderful children, Taylor and Kyle, for your patience as I took time away from you to work on this project.

My sister, whose loving support I'll always cherish.

My mother, without whose example of caring, love, and strength I would not have been able to continue the work my father began, in our practice and on this book.

Everyone who reads this book; I hope the advice that you find here will make a big difference in your lives.

Dad, I would be nothing without you.

INDEX

Page numbers in *italic* indicate illustrations.

www.thetruthaboutbackpainbook.com

Be part of the growing community of thousands who have discovered the joys of living without back pain. Log on to:

- Learn more about the Arch, the product uniquely designed to give you the best results in back opening and optimal stretching. This is the product I developed personally and use in my practice every day.

- Sign up for the free *Balance in the Body* newsletters that will provide you with tips, treatments, and reminders to living back-pain-free each and every day.

- Download recipes specifically developed with the Structural/Nutritional/Emotional philosophy in mind for healing and wellness.

About the Authors

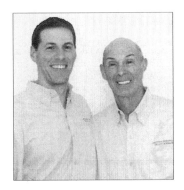

Dr. Todd Sinett is the owner of the Midtown Chiropractic Health and Wellness practice in New York City (www.midtownchiro.com), which provides chiropractic care and applied kinesiology, nutritional and supportive counseling, and physical and massage therapy to thousands of individuals, including noted sports figures and celebrities. The center hosts weekend wellness programs and corporate informational seminars as well as publishing a periodic online newsletter, *Balance in the Body* (www.balanceinthebody.com). Sinett is a recognized expert in chiropractic and applied kinesiology and has served as clinical expert for many television programs including *The View*, *FoxMD*, and *Good Day New York*. His website is www.drsinett.com.

For more than forty years, **Dr. Sheldon Sinett** was a leading chiropractor and a pioneer in combining chiropractic medicine with a variety of cutting-edge, holistic practices.

31901050572413